AF822552

The New Royal Rife Book

Physics Study Says Royal Rife's Claims "Experimentally Confirmed"

Barry Lynes

ISBN: 978-1-7337645-2-0

Published by:
BioMed Publishing Group, LLC
PO BOX 550531
South Lake Tahoe CA 96155

To order additional copies of this book and see our selection of Rife-related books & DVDs, please visit:

www.BioMedPublishers.com

Disclaimer: This books' contents is not professional medical advice nor should it be used as such. For all medical conditions, consult a licensed medical practitioner. This book is intended for educational and informational purposes only, and does not substitute for professional medical advice or consultation with healthcare professionals

Interview of Dr. Richard Gerber, author of *Vibrational Medicine*. By Edward Brown at website share-international.org (SI).

SI: "Can you tell our readers what exactly vibrational medicine is?"

Dr. Gerber: "Vibrational medicine is a diagnostic and healing approach to illness using energy in various forms and frequencies. As a therapy, vibrational medicine is the application of different types of energy for healing ... In some ways I see vibrational medicine as an evolving sub-specialty of medicine."

SI: "I was wondering if you were familiar with the work of Royal Rife, with his universal microscope and the treatment of cancer with energy frequencies?

Dr. Gerber: "Rife is just now beginning to become known for his work with cancer therapy ... The Rife beam ray seemed to be extremely effective in treating cancer ... The potential of non-invasive energy medicine to benefit people at a much lower cost is phenomenal."

Royal Rife

"A USC clinical research study with 16 terminally-ill cancer patient took place in 1934. Rife insisted that a panel of medical experts supervise the study in which he used his Beam Ray instrument to destroy the cancer-causing organisms. The medical staff pronounced fourteen of the sixteen patients in the study clinically cured after 70 days. The other two required 20 more days of medical treatment before they, too, were well."

Jule Klotter, *Townsend Letter for Doctors* January 2004

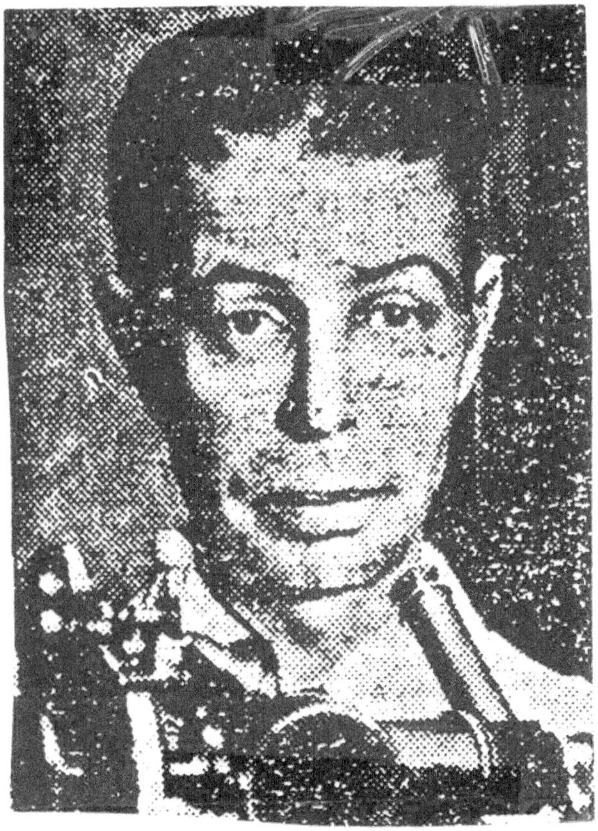

Royal Rife as a young scientist

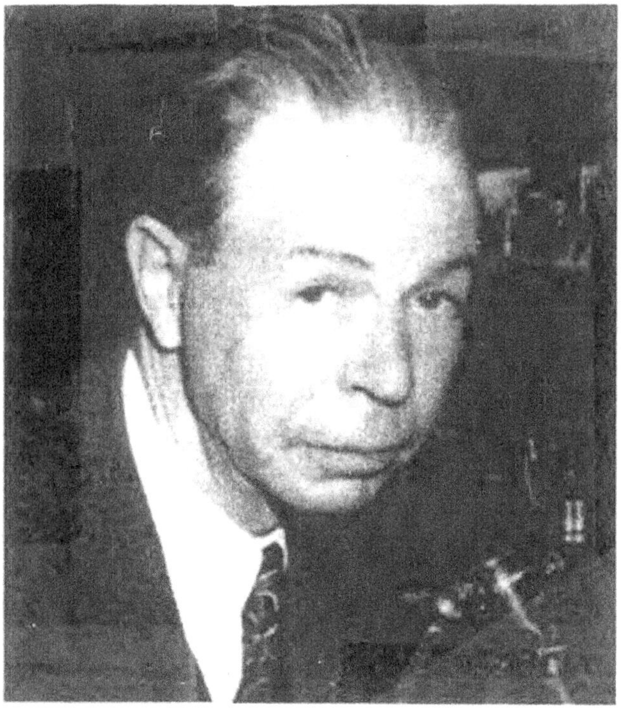

Royal Rife as a mature scientist

Science Triumph -- Royal Rife Returns

Sometimes in history a special person comes along who provides monumental discoveries that alter forever science and medicine. Royal Rife was such a person and he did something extraordinary. He showed the world the hidden regions of disease, making possible the first steps toward a new medicine.

His genius with microscopes opened the way to viewing what never before had been seen. Like Galileo with his telescope, Royal Rife with his microscope started something that may carry us far.

This book contains many voices which will tell the reader about the life and work of Royal Rife. It also explains in plain language the marvelous breakthroughs that resulted from his experiments with light, frequencies, resonance, and the diligent "mapping" of the micro world! Rife created a "color table" for every pathogen, where each disease-causing microorganism had a unique, ordered place. The healing possibilities resulting from this groundbreaking register are enormous.

Further, this book illuminates a direction our modern scientists, health practitioners, and public health policymakers need to explore that may enable many millions to be healed of various ailments or simply to realize a constant state of optimal health.

"... these waves, or this ray, as the frequencies might be called, have been shown to possess the power of devitalizing disease organisms ... when tuned to an exact wave length, or frequency, for each different organism."

Royal Rife (1888-1971)
Microscopist & Microbiologist
The Evening Tribune, San Diego, May 6, 1938

"Royal Rife ... examined cancers with the optical microscopes which he designed and built ... he then designed electrical machines which he could tune to certain frequencies and apparently cause the viruses to disintegrate as he observed them with his microscope."

Peter Macomber, M.D., Harvard-trained
pathologist and former Chief of
Experimental Pathology at Walter Reed
Army Institute of Pathology, Washington,
D.C., from *Townsend Letter for Doctors*
October 1994

"... it was my presumption that when the causative agent of malignancy would be found, it would be found to be caused by a micro-organism. Not unlikely a so-called non-pathogenic micro-organism which we have with us at all times. The etiology of this theoretical and applied biology can no longer be denied and I have demonstrated it time and again."

"A Discussion on Laboratory Research"
by Royal R. Rife (June 14, 1958)

"The real voyage of discovery consists not in seeking new landscapes, but in having new eyes."

Marcel Proust (1871-1922)
Insightful French author

Royal Rife gave us new eyes. The world he explored and the discoveries he made led to an original method to heal many human diseases. We are stupid, obstructive, and corrupt as a society if we do not insist on a rigorous, comprehensive, and independent program that tests Rife frequency medicine. There is sufficient proof that it will cure many, if not all, microbe-caused diseases!

Today's versions of Rife's resonance instruments can be easily integrated into modern clinical practices once the public gains knowledge of its awesome potential -- to painlessly, noninvasively eliminate deadly diseases. We must not let orthodox medicine continue a scandalous suppression of a world-changing biophysics technology.

Lots of people already use Rife devices, which are being created in many places around the globe. The further development of this evolutionary health advance needs only time for Rife's conclusive results to overcome resistance.

Rife made historic medical science discoveries because his super microscope invention gave the world "new eyes!" Then he found the elegant potency of <u>resonance healing</u>.

D

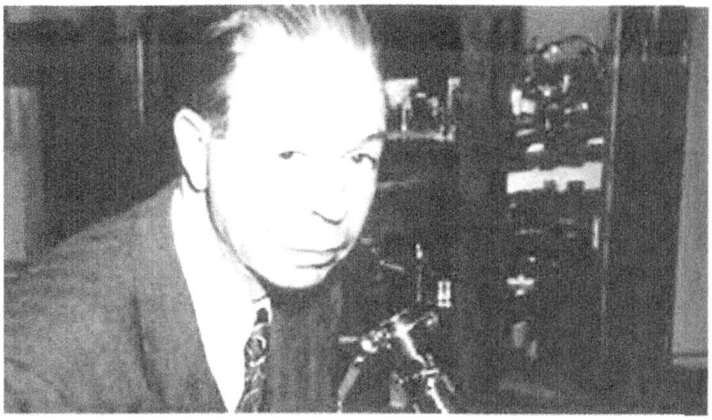

Royal Rife Takes A Bow

Top Scientist Declares Rife's Discovery "Experimentally Confirmed" – Physics Journal Tells Science Community Of Effective Healing Technology

E

The New Royal Rife Book

by Barry Lynes

A Compilation and Transformative Creative Work which may benefit public understanding of the profound curative potential of BioPhysics. This discovery of "resonance healing" may be a very effective method for curing painlessly and noninvasively <u>microbe-caused diseases.</u> All because of the research, discoveries, and inventions of Royal Raymond Rife (1888-1971).

F

Who was Royal Rife?

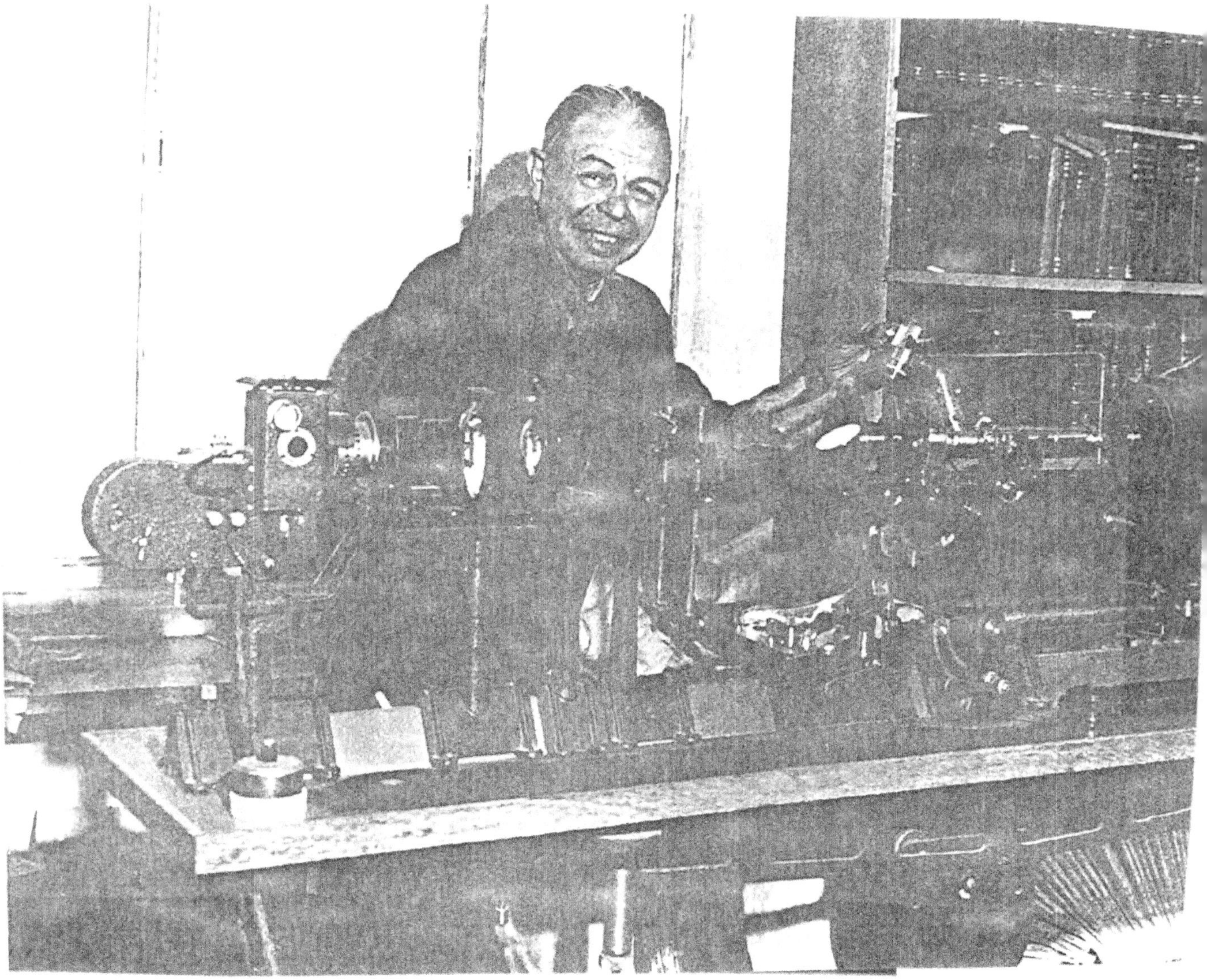

And what did he do that scared the money powers into bribing and intimidating scientists and doctors to stop endorsing and using Rife's profound scientific and medical discoveries?

There is a tale to be told if the mainstream journalists ever regained their professional courage and integrity.

Contents

H

Part I

A Physicist's Document Validates Royal Rife's Profound Science Contribution To BioPhysics Cures Of Deadly Diseases

"Virus Destruction by Resonance" by Auguste Meessen, from December 2020 issue of *Journal of Modern Physics* Link:

https//www.scirp.org/journal/paperinformation.aspx?paperid=106157

Part 1. Meessen Says Rife's Theory Is Experimentally Confirmed

In 1933, Royal Rife invented the world's greatest optical microscope. He called it the "Universal" microscope. It achieved enormous magnification and superior resolution, enabling him to view living, virus-sized microbes for the first time in the history of microbiology! Royal Rife broke "the vision barrier" established by German physicist Ernst Abbe in 1873!

This wonderful invention enabled Royal Rife to see organisms of the micro-world never studied previously. It also allowed him to experiment with the causes of humanity's deadliest diseases. So he began researching a previously hidden world where he discovered a revolutionary method of healing! Rife learned that each microbe -- bacteria, virus, nanobacteria -- had a unique oscillatory rate. Once he identified this "signature" frequency, he could destroy the cause of a particular disease by intensifying that frequency until the microbe either exploded or gathered into a lifeless clump. This opened a door to a painless, noninvasive method to cure human diseases! All because his super microscope gave him "new eyes" to view living, virus-sized microbes!

Eventually this exciting scientific breakthrough had a totally unexpected and terrible effect on Royal Rife's life. He was perceived as an immediate threat and competitive foe of the financial interests that dominated medicine. So the established medical powers suppressed Royal Rife's amazingly efficient therapy that cured deadly diseases! Even though it had proved to be 100% successful in curing 16 "hopeless" cancer patients in a 1934 clinical trial sponsored by the University of Southern California. Royal Rife's therapy was an unexpected and disconcerting futuristic technology that disrupted the cozy world of orthodox medicine and Royal Rife himself was soon considered to be the "dangerous genius of San Diego!" Just as Nikola Tesla had once been perceived by electric companies as a threat to their oligopoly power and profits.

In 1937 or 1938, the boss of the American Medical Association (AMA) learned of Royal Rife's fantastic electronic cures for deadly diseases. This medical politician soon sought "to buy in" to Rife's Beam Ray company which built the frequency devices that were bringing patients some fantastic cures.

The AMA boss – Dr. Morris Fishbein – was a known shakedown artist who promoted worthless drugs if their makers paid him the high advertising fees he demanded for the AMA's monthly journal. So now "the kingpin of American Medicine" (according to Associated Press science writer Howard Blakeslee) was trying to take over Rife's new electro-medicine therapy. Except Royal Rife refused to let the AMA's corrupt boss be in charge of a "pure science" revolution or natural science phenomenon.

But Rife's refusal to allow the AMA boss to determine how this revolution in medicine would be integrated into medical practices only increased Fishbein's determination to obtain Rife's oscillatory instrument by other means – by crime. So the AMA boss bribed Rife's engineer to sell out Rife and with an AMA-paid attorney, seek to legally steal the Beam Ray company. Rife and the other partners just didn't comprehend the kind of opponent they faced. Or what length Fishbein would go to abuse the political power of his position as head of the AMA!

A year-long trial in 1939 resulted in the AMA boss losing his attempt at legal theft. But the trial ruined Royal Rife. His "Beam Ray" company was made bankrupt and Rife became an alcoholic. Fishbein then imposed a total prohibition on Rife's science discovery and "resonance" therapy! One of the foulest deeds in the long history of American medicine soon unfolded, causing immeasurable pain and tragedy for scores of millions of cancer sufferers for the next 8 decades!

The AMA headquarters sent out an order that all doctors who used Rife's Beam Ray frequency device would lose their license to practice medicine! Plus a brutal censorship was put into effect on Rife. This lasted from 1940 to 2020!

2020 – The Revolutionary Article

Until 2020 when a PHYSICS journal broke the censorship wall. Because of one man – Auguste Meessen, emeritus professor of physics at the Catholic University of Louvan (Belgium). Meessen had studied under George Lemaitre (Father of the Big Bang theory) and taught for many years the most complicated realms of physics. As a full professor, he taught Quantum Mechanics, Theoretical Physics, Solid State Physics, and Didactics for physics teachers. He was a scholar who turned his sophisticated physics knowledge to the prohibited topic of Royal Rife, Rife's supermicroscope, and Rife's discovery that disease could be healed using resonance frequencies!

In December 2020, Professor of Physics Auguste Meessen broke the EIGHT

DECADES of censorship of Rife's science accomplishments by establishment medicine and establishment science. Professor Meessen informed the scientific community that Rife's "scientific creativity and accomplished craftsmanship deserved recognition and respect." AMA's cruel corruption was exposed!

A top scholar and physics professor -- Auguste Meessen -- had just published an article that praised Royal Rife's long suppressed discovery of healing disease by resonance! Because Rife's supermicroscope actually did what the scientific community believed was impossible -- see living, virus-sized microbes that caused humanity's deadliest diseases. And because Rife had found a way to destroy the disease causes, Meessen's article revealed the political motives behind the attacks against Rife's therapy. The medical elite was being accused of an inexcusable suppression of a viable cure for many ailments!

What the mainstream media and the scientific journals dared not tell, Auguste Meessen openly discussed. He broke the censorship wall and challenged honest scientists to look at what was revealed in the December 2020 *Journal of Modern Physics*. Professor of Physics Auguste Meessen's 41-page article titled "Virus Destruction by Resonance" explained the laws of physics and provided the equations which confirmed that Royal Rife's long-suppressed achievement was, indeed, scientifically valid!

Professor Meessen declared, "These supermicroscopes allowed him (Rife) to make extraordinary discoveries, but they contradicted the beliefs of medical authorities." That was what organized medicine had deceitfully done for 80 years. Caused horrible pain and death for personal profit and power!

A legitimate discovery of enormous importance that the medical community should have been delighted to develop and use, instead had been suppressed! Which prevented patients having a ***noninvasive*** option for healing their misery. Meessen had publicly said a great wrong resulted from medical dogma and abuse of the AMA's political power.

Rife's method for healing was opposed primarily by the Drug Trust! Not because of poor science, but to protect the financial interests of medical doctors and drug manufacturers! The AMA's self-serving censoring had been openly exposed! The "scientific community" had been informed by Auguste Meessen that modern physics laws revealed why Rife's therapy was worthy of respect and recognition! Which meant it should be developed and used by patients with microbe-caused diseases. Including cancer, the sacred cash cow of medicine, government, and Wall Street's largest portfolios.

This was a scandal of the first order. Comparable to the Vatican's treatment of Galileo and the forbidden Sun-centered concept so many centuries before! With Rife, the medical establishment was guilty of an outrageous obstruction of a major scientific advance which threatened traditional medicine and its ruling chemotherapy product. Rife's discoveries could disrupt many existing medical, scientific, and financial "interests" and for that reason, these power centers pressured and bribed Rife's science associates to force them to abandon Rife and the "resonance" approach to healing (biophysics).

Meessen wrote that the Nobel Prize in chemistry had been awarded in 2014 to scientists making notable advances in "super-resolved microscopy" just as Royal Rife's supermicroscope already had achieved in the early 1930s! But Meessen emphasized that the modern scientists had used lasers to achieve their goals; while Rife had done something equal or better using classical means. Yet Royal Rife had been erased from history because of the AMA's enmity.

Meessen: "The Nobel Prize in Chemistry of 2014 was actually awarded for the development of *super-resolved microscopy*. This was achieved by using powerful lasers, while Rife succeeded with purely classical means ... his name has been wiped out from official medicine and scientific literature." (Underlining added.)

Meessen was disgusted that high officials could do such harm to society for such ignoble motives. Meessen wrote that the suppression of alternative medicine by Big Pharma and doctor associations were despicable deeds. And that they kept actual cures from people learning they existed! Meessen recognized that the cost of such misconduct was deadly.

Meessen: "It is necessary to realize that it was profoundly unjust, unscientific and even harmful, by preventing possible cure." Blunt and focused, Meessen was condemning the medicine and science autocrats who had done such a thing against ethical principles and the good of society!

What Auguste Meessen also did with his defiant refusal to stay quiet about a science and medical censorship was legitimize discussion of Rife's inventions and important microbiological discoveries. No longer could AMA officials and other traditional medicine authorities simply tell the lie that Rife had been disproved. Now Rife's amazing findings and new therapy for healing diseases had a top scientific mind explaining the physics that provided a foundation for Rife's revolutionary biophysics or frequency therapy!

Professor of Physics Auguste Meessen openly stated in his long, detailed 41-page article that the world had a biophysics method which should be recognized in treating serious diseases because it deserved to be recognized just as biochemical treatments now were!

Meessen: "It would ... be irresponsible to neglect already existing evidence that an efficient, safe and rapidly adaptable biophysical method is possible." (Underlining added.)

Bravo to Professor Meessen for saying what so many in the "professional" science and medical worlds dared not say! Where had the young hotshots of science and medicine of previous generations been? Those who avoided Rife and would not conduct honest investigations of Rife's microscope or his healing through frequency destruction of a disease's cause? They had ducked in order to advance their careers – at the expense of patients, ethical codes, and the greater public health interest of recognizing and developing with resources and personnel something of great value to the "healing arts"!

Meessen: "Rife's method could have been tested at least by means of experimental procedures, but it was rejected since it seemed to be unbelievable. Nevertheless, it is also necessary to explain why the reported facts are true." And Professor Meessen certainly did! He explained for his physics peers why Rife's discoveries work, using the modern understanding of physics laws! In very complicated, advanced physics language and diagrams!

Which eventually may lead to modern medicine being honest with the public! Censorship and suppression of a brilliant breakthrough healing therapy can no longer be ignored! Because such deliberate wrong could mean death to innocent patients. The abuse of power by organized medicine can no longer hide the reality that some diseases can be cured by resonance – destroying the microbe cause of a disease, reversing the disease condition as Royal Rife did in the 1930s, and in time, curing many patients by using this finally recognized biophysics method!

Meesen: "Rife's method is not dangerous at all and efficient for destroying virulent microbes anywhere inside our body. Rife discovered ... that bacteria and nanobacteria can be destroyed by resonance." Wow. That is clearly what the AMA, the American Cancer Society, and the National Cancer Institute did not want known and had worked so hard to keep from the American people. By totally ignoring their responsibility to society of guarding and telling the truth, not hiding it in order to personally gain money or position or security.

Meessen: "Rife was able to see exploding nanobacteria ... He did then prove that some of them are present in cancer tissue and that after being cultured, they do cause cancer. He (Rife) determined the resonant frequency for targeted destruction of various microbes. These values were confirmed by two collaborators, using different equipment."

In other words, independent scientific tests confirmed the validity of Rife's original research! Rife's work had never been "disproved", as the American Cancer Society (ACS) so blatantly fabricated!

Meessen was the best advocate for Royal Rife that had ever existed! His power came from his knowledge, not a high position in the AMA or at a government agency or within a private cancer center. Where a conflict of interest tainted any denouncement of Royal Rife's revolutionary approach to curing cancer and many other diseases! (Rife found the "signature" frequency for the microbial causes of approximately 50 diseases!) Yet the AMA and the FDA and others had buried it all while being totally ignorant of its truth because none of them bothered to do an honest investigation. Just followed orders. Which resulted in truly horrendous death counts.

Snooty modern academics still complain that Rife's work can't be found in elite "peer-reviewed" science and medical publications! Of course not. The AMA thoroughly prevented such studies and evidence being published! Thus the absence of such articles as the academics complain about only prove the AMA's treachery, not Rife's lack of scientific ability.

Meessen then introduced the subject of the successful 1934 clinical trial using frequency to heal cancer by destroying the BX nanobacteria cause!

Meessen: "The efficiency of his method for healing cancer was clinically tested, but even those results were declared to be bogus since they required modifying cherished postulates. For those who had the power to crush Rife, it did not matter that the reported results might be true. Rife was prosecuted. His documents were stolen. Instruments were wrecked ... his achievements were eradicated from official medical record. That was profoundly unjust, truly antiscientific and detrimental for the worldwide health system."

So organized vindictiveness came at Royal Rife in the late 1930s and afterwards because he threatened the medical monopoly by discovering something better than what they had.

Meessen: "Rife made a great discovery. We did only explain why apparently unbelievable, but observable facts are true. Now it is up to other persons and institutions to carry on."

Meessen: "It was a huge error to claim that the observed facts had to be bogus, without verifying, since it deprived humanity from use of a simple and secure method to fight sicknesses, plagues and even cancer."

Meessen: "The theory is experimentally confirmed and leaves no rational reason to negate the possibility of targeted destruction of microbes."

Meessen: "We have to insist that dogmatism and concentration of power endanger scientific progress by blocking freedom of thought."

Meessen: "Rife mentioned ... that the BX entities (microbe cause of cancer) are actively moving around, but that he found a method to 'devitalize' all microorganisms as desired. It required EM waves of particular frequency, depending on the kind of microbes. This frequency was determined by observing the microbes with his microscope."

Meessen: "After Rife's trial, orchestrated already in 1939 by AMA, he was forced to stop his research. He was bankrupt and desperate. His laboratory had been raided. His microscopes were made unusable and documents were stolen."

Thus the "Great Silence" was broken. For 8 1/2 decades since the 1934 clinical trial which proved Royal Rife's resonance therapy for cancer brought 100% cures, the medical establishment had kept that truth hidden so it could teach medical students its Pharma medicine and not allow them to know about a super alternative therapy that patients should have "the right to try." Thank God the world still occasionally has people such as Auguste Meessen!

Ugly "Cancer Research" World

For many decades the orthodox oncologists (cancer specialists) at the National Cancer Instiute (NCI) and their affiliated researchers at colleges or private cancer centers protected the virtual monopoly of chemotherapy! Any potential treatment which might have threatened Big Pharma's profits was institutionally killed. This clever sabotage of dozens of alternatives, ultimately numbering 100 or more was a secret attack on any non-drug cancer therapy.

When the "alternative" treatments gained limited recogniton after 1991 (OAM, NCCAM, NCCIH)), the "deep state" of cancer bureaucrats and "defenders of Chemo" immediately killed the attempt to have "Field Tests" -- where government science investigators destroyed the unanimous decision to travel to sites worldwide where alternative methods were obtaining good results, and then initiate clinical trials of these innovative therapies. The defenders of orthodoxy had to kill such a threat! So they imposed a different agenda! Spend that grant money instead at elite universities and have "academics" study these "crazy" alternatives! They killed the field studies by trusting the professional medical scientists. Who were already being bribed by Big Pharma! The "field" concept was completely buried! Top doctors who received payoffs from Big Pharma also were allowed to veto anything about which they had negative views. Which was the final "Kiss of Death."

The result? Chemo remained dominant. Any alternative with a good record and growing interest by honest practitioners was quietly blocked or NCI trials were rigged to fail. Pharma kept its profits high! And any internet researcher today will find NOTHING – no honest "history of the secret suppression of alternative cancer therapies." They will find lots of articles by the government's "complementary" and "alternative" and "integrative" (CAM) specialists who – in unison – do declare that "alternative cancer therapies don't work and are dangerous." Almost complete 100% agreement on that! Because the "fix" was in from the start. Thus unnecessary suffering and death came to cancer victims who had no approved alternatives. (No "Right to Try" for them!) So much for citizen liberty in determining what should be done with one's own body as even the Supreme Court has declared a sacred legal principle!

All because the professional "cancer experts" make so much money by "researching" what their Pharma paymasters want! Of course the media avoids certain subjects. Pharma pays the media huge advertising fees to stay away from investigating Pharma's role in suppressing alternative therapies. Not just Royal Rife's "resonance" therapy. So the "free press" does not report why chemo remains the "standard of practice" and supposedly "science based" method for anyone who has cancer! With 100 alternative therapies chosen by the US government's "alternative agency" to be fairly tested. But never were because of medical politics,

So it makes no sense to continue spending billions of dollars annually for a National Cancer Institute (NCI) filled with corrupt pharma servants! Who refused to conduct honest tests of safe, non-toxic cancer therapies!

Just don't expect them to reveal how they sabotaged those tests. The truth is told in quotations HERE in this book! Especially those on PAGE 29, PAGE 38, PAGE 40, PAGE 53, PAGE 57, PAGE 66, and PAGE 67! The public wasn't informed why the "field trials" were canceled! Cancer experts used various maneuvers to avoid what the alternative medicine agency was set up to do! NCI chose to ignore the public.

The basic understanding of what makes a "Rife Machine" succeed is known. A number of modern engineers did the "sleuthing" by sharing information in a cooperative effort to "save" Rife's great gift to humanity.

The BEAM RAY #5 device from 1937-1939 obtained fantastic and reliable results. Until the AMA stopped it from being built by forcing its makers into court for a year long ordeal, bankrupting the BEAM RAY company, and then ordering all physicians who were getting incredible healing from Rife's BEAM RAY to surrender their new electronic device that destroyed the causes of microbial diseases. Or lose their licenses to practice medicine!

"What if a health crime against humanity tribunal were convened ... in the enlightened future and those who had pushed ... against alternative medicine – those who deny patients information about and access to less expensive, safe, and nontoxic treatments – were on trial for such actions? ... doctors and administrators ... needlessly costing lives ... millions in the past 100 years have died of cancer ... with the toxic residues of chemotherapy agents in their blood. What I am asking is merely an exercise. One day it will no longer be an exercise; it will be a real accounting."

"Cancer and Health Crimes Against Humanity" by Burton Goldberg nfam.org.

From *The Microscopist* by Paul Dunbar
at website thelethaltext.me (April 24, 2018)
(All Underlining added for emphasis.)

"The suppression of Nikola Tesla sets the tone for the management of science in the twentieth century ... Three decades after the banks moved on Tesla, it all happened again, this time to the microscopist Royal Rife, who can justly be called the Tesla of microbiology. Rife, like Tesla, combined scientific insight with extraordinary skill in engineering. With Rife, as with Tesla, new technology was suppressed ... the bacteria with life frequency equal to the frequency the Rife machine was set, would start to resonate, and just like a glass that breaks when it's hit by the right frequency, the bacteria would die.

"... Rife was able to prove his findings to anyone who dared to see through his amazing microscope. His attackers never saw through his microscope ... The same happened to Galileo who claimed that the Sun was the center of our solar system and not the earth. He was ridiculed and nobody would even look through his telescope to observe the proof.

"The science of microbiology had always been distanced from its object first by the limits of our senses and then by the limits of our optical technology.

"When these limits were shattered by the optical engineer Roy Rife, the medical establishment ... shut him down, drove him out of his country, and prosecuted any of his followers who did not abjure the heretic.

"The rest they left to the power of forgetting.

"Rife ... continued his work ... in 1932 he was able to isolate a microbe that is present in all cancers. He called it BX -- Bacillus X -- virus and gave it the formal name of Cryptocides Primordiates, 'hidden primordial killer'. Like all microbes, it was pleomorphic, manifesting four different forms, depending on its environment.

"The medical establishment reacted like a medieval trade guild protecting its secrets, and ruthlessly suppressed Rife's work, his company, and his technology ... We went back to a microbiology of corpses and empty shells.

"Like Tesla, Rife was taken down at his peak, and by the time the world

had gone through another long and hideous global war, it was as it he had never existed. Like Tesla, he was written out of the history books and is largely forgotten. The first man to see a live virus, the isolator of the cancer virus, and the inventor of the cure -- a man whose name should be immortal -- forgotten. Written out.

"This was no war of ideas, but naked violence perpetrated in defense of an outdated paradigm on behalf of the corporations and financial interests behind pharmaceutical medicine. Pay-offs and threats, bribery and blackmail, confiscation of equipment, sabotage, theft, arson and, above all, the AMA's threat to withdraw medical licenses, crushed the movement among doctors. Finally, regulations controlling the use of radio frequencies was introduced, making Rife's machines effectively illegal.

"Thus Western medicine is based – deliberately and knowingly so since Rife – on an incomplete theory of disease causation. Pasteur's monomorphism, like wire-based electronic transmission, delivered a straight-forward and profitable business model: for every disease is a germ; for every germ a pill or vaccine. The entire pharmacuetical industry and the medical profession it controls are built on these myopic monomorphic principles.

"Cancer in the post-war era was built into a terrifying monster, but it was protected by a bigger monster, the corporations who profit from its simulated treatment, and their agents within the public institutions who pursue and persecute anyone -- and there have been many -- who developed a cure.

"This is not a health system, but a business model masquerading as one.

"And then, in the immediate post-war years, the final, sick joke in the cancer treatment: chemotherapy."

"The Universal Microscope"

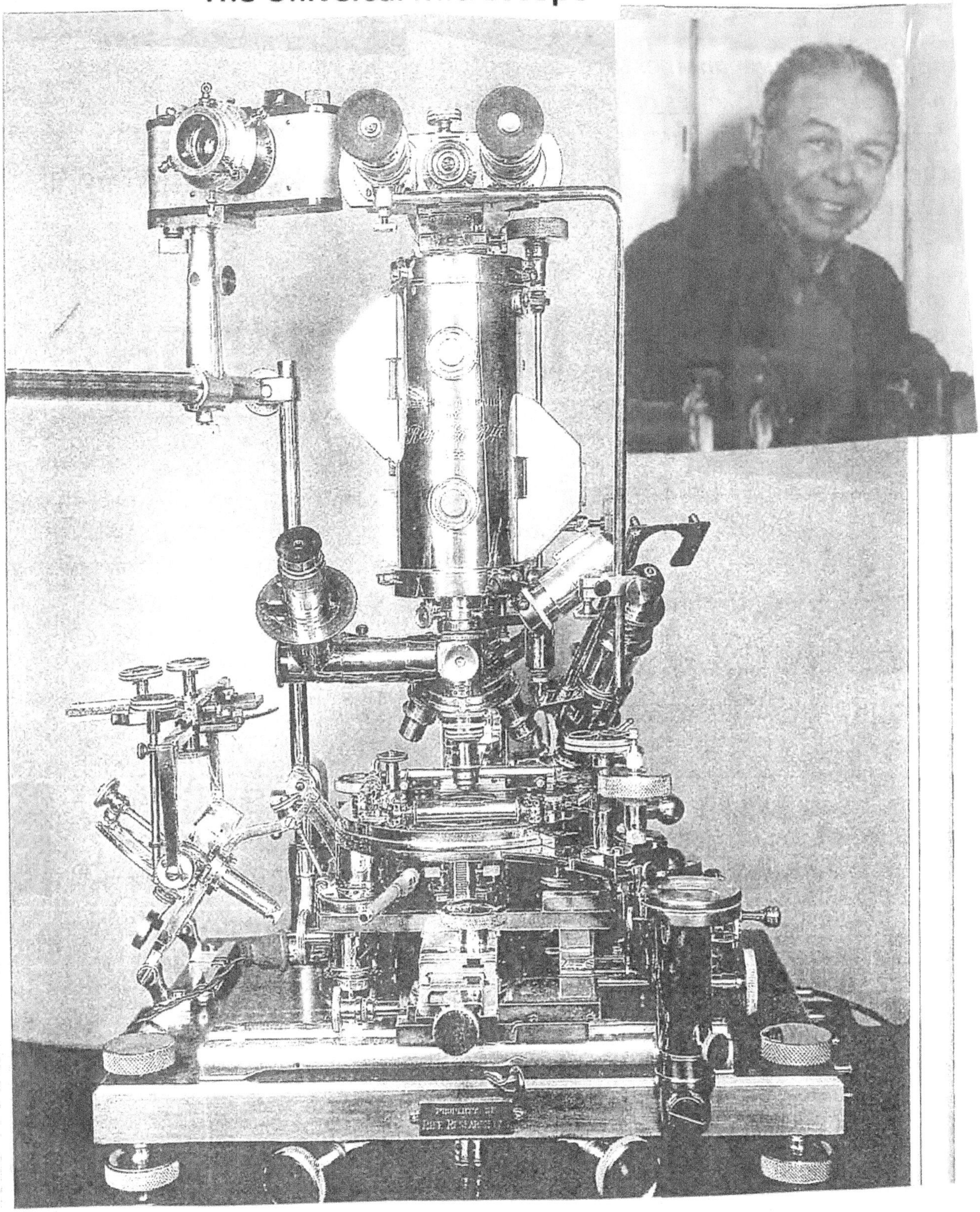

Royal Rife

"I believe this instrument will open fields that have never been seen before by the human eye."

Royal Rife

Royal Rife -- 1930's lab & Newspaper Headline 1938

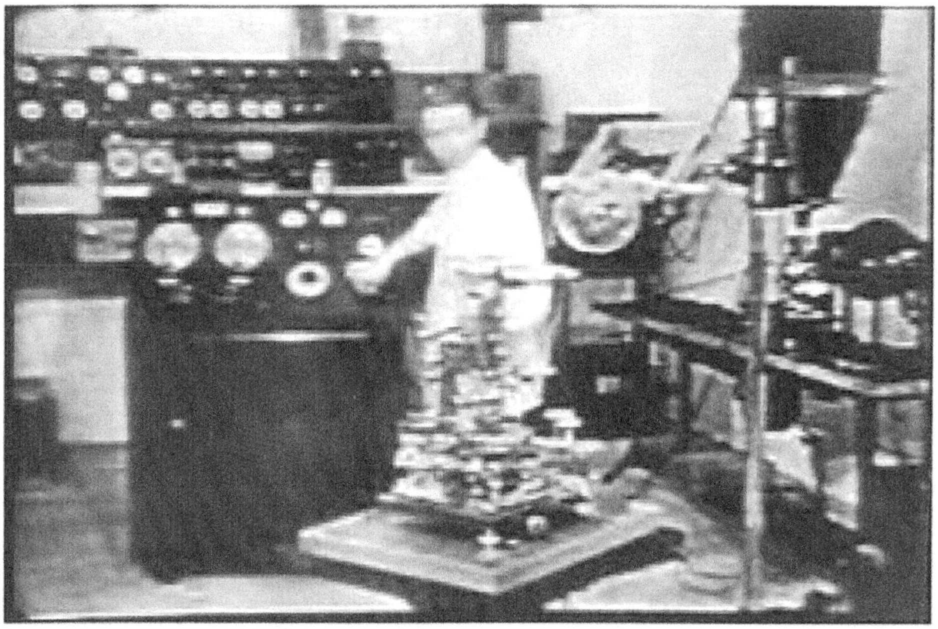

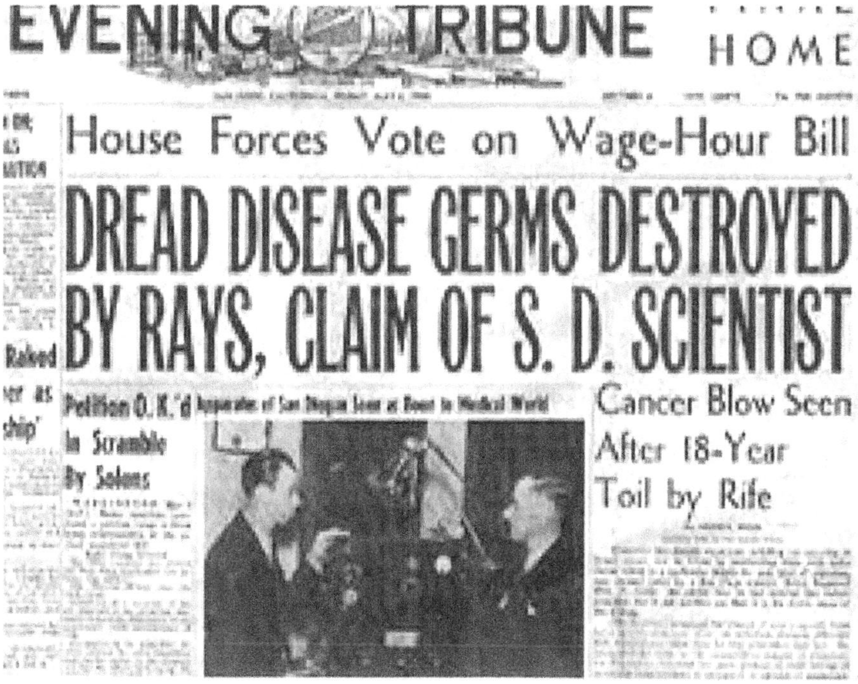

EVENING TRIBUNE HOME

House Forces Vote on Wage-Hour Bill

DREAD DISEASE GERMS DESTROYED BY RAYS, CLAIM OF S. D. SCIENTIST

Petition O.K.'d In Scramble By Solons

Cancer Blow Seen After 18-Year Toil by Rife

"Rife's microscope played no role in the actual destruction of the pathogenic organism, but it allowed him to view the effects of the electric fields from the Beam Ray tube upon the organism itself."

"Forbidden Cures"
educateyourself.org

"Scientific Marvel"

"But of all of his scientific marvels, the intricately built microscope, culmination of two decades development, seems the greatest."

Los Angeles Times, June 26, 1940

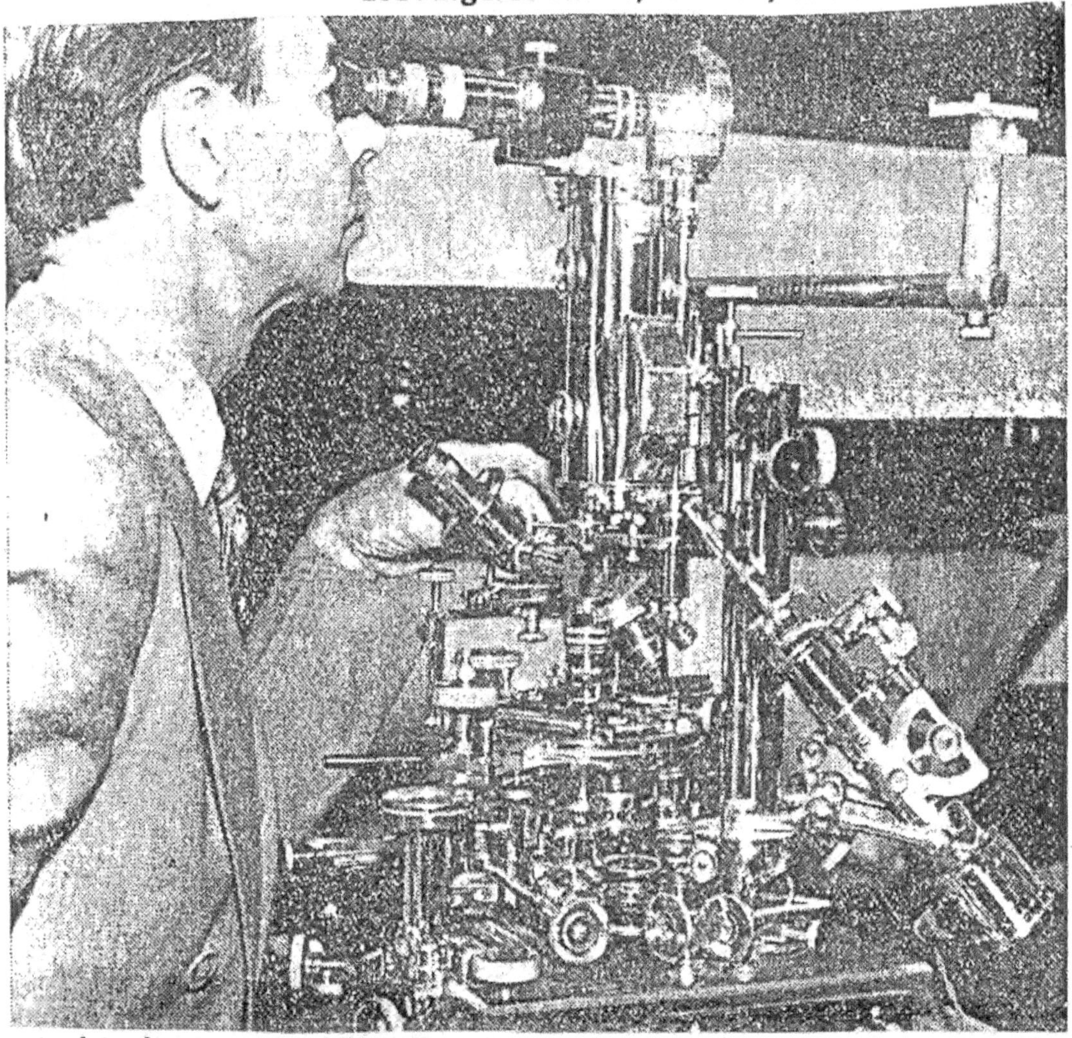

Reported to be so powerful that it reveals disease organisms never seen before, the giant microscope pictured above has just been completed by Royal R. Rife, of San Diego, Calif, whose home-built instruments have long been ranked among the finest in the world. To eliminate distortion, the image produced by the new two-foot-tall apparatus does not pass through the usual air-filled tube, but along an optical path of quartz blocks and prisms. Weighing 200 pounds, the microscope has 5,682 parts.

Los Angles Times OCTOBER 1940

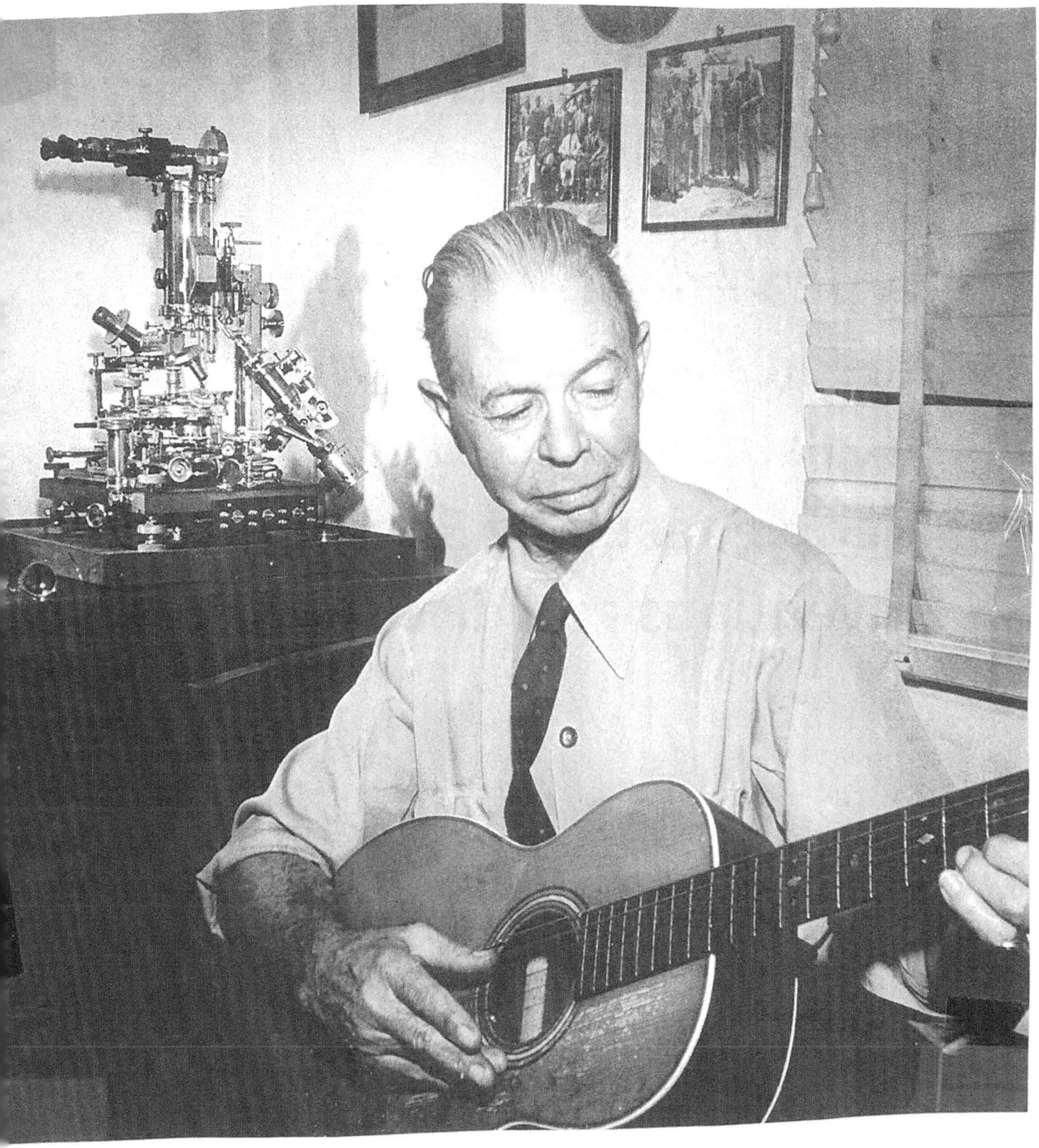

Royal Rife relaxing with guitar. The Rife Universal Microscope stands on a table in the left background.

Part II

A penetrating 14-page study of medical science knowledge explained to us by smart people teaching Royal Rife's inventions and discoveries.

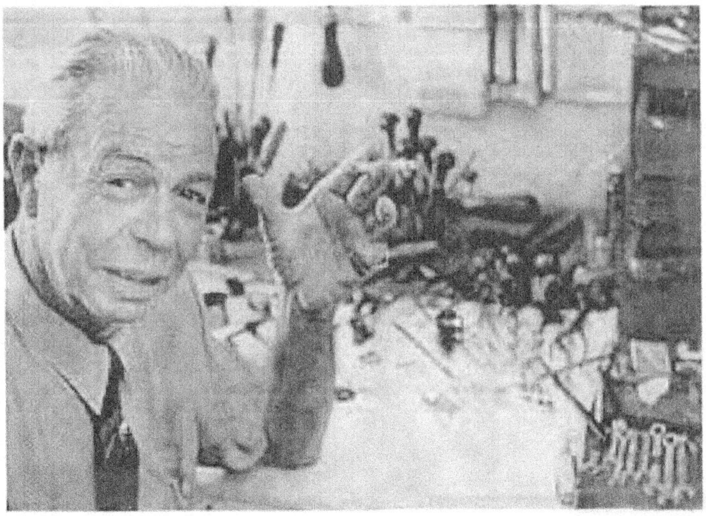

Royal Rife sends a greeting to future generations (us!)

Part II. A Penetrating Study of Royal Rife's Wizardry

How did Royal R. Rife -- a science researcher and microscope inventor -- determine the frequency that would destroy a specific microbe that caused a known (or unknown) disease? He watched through his microscope a microbe that caused a specific disease -- such as the rod form bacteria that caused tuberculosis -- and then tried one frequency after another for extended periods until he found the specific frequency that destroyed that bacteria! His way of searching and finding the "killer" frequency also worked with the "filter-passing forms" of virus size. What today microbiologists call "nanobacteria". Without his supermicroscope that enabled him to watch if any frequency effected the tiny micro-organism, there was no way to determine the frequency that would destroy the bacteria, nanobacteria, fungi or virus and cure the disease associated with a specific microbe. Here's how Royal Rife himself explained what he did:

"We simply hunt and try. That was all we could do. We could put a pure culture of the organism under the microscope and I start in and I tune this thing until I find a frequency that will destroy it." (Rife's voice recorded on tape in the 1950s.)

The Rise and Fall of a Scientific Genius (2007)
a video by Shawn Montgomery at zerozerotwo.org

After Rife isolated his BX cancer virus, he used it to heal cancer:

"He discovered that at a specific frequency, the rays would lead to explosion and destruction of BX viruses. When the viruses were destroyed, the cancer tumor slowly reduced and ultimately disappeared within a couple of months. Cancer was cured."

"Is Cancer Caused By A Virus?
By Arvind Kulkarni, Radio oncologist, USA
Bombay Hospital Journal 2002
website bhi.org.in/journal/2002

"Tuning the turning dial near the specimen, he would know the lethal setting ... Soon a catalogue of lethal pitches would be amassed. With this Dr. Rife could wage victorious wars against every disease in existence." (Underlining added.)

"Royal Raymond Rife & His Amazing Micoscope"
by Gerry Vassilatos at unariumwisdom.com

"Let us look at the most unknown, and most suppressed therapy of all, Rife frequencies.

"RIFE: Rife, after its inventor, Dr. Royal Rife, may be considered a subdivision of electronic medicine, yet in reality is more based on ultra-sound. Dr. Rife himself, not being a physicist, can be forgiven for not completely understanding the actual nature of his device. In general, Rife can be considered to be a resonant frequency-based therapy, those frequencies being generated in any number of ways but being essentially ultrasound upon hitting the dead skin layer." (Underlining added.)

"Alternatives to Surgery and Drugs"
by John Q. Citizen
Updated 2015
ahm -- portal.com/Alternatives

"The key to fighting cancer and other diseases successfully lies in the potential of destroying the pathogenic microorganisms and getting the body to excrete them. The microbial activity is the basis for the growth process of the tumor.

"The remedies can heal the individual at any stage in the growth process if the microbial process is reversed." (Underlining added.)

Advanced Microscopy for Nutritional Evaluation and Correction (1997)
by Michael Coyle, Ph.D.

"Royal Rife ... was a well known scientist because of his breakthrough invention of an extremely powerful microscope and he was very successful in curing certain diseases. He was highly regarded within the scientific community until the medical establishment came down on him and erased him from history ... the threat to orthodox medicine was too great. Medical officials and societies mounted a furious counterattack against Rife's monumental discovery before the American public could be informed of it. One of the greatest scientific and medical discoveries of the 20th century was ruthlessly shoved into a dungeon of history."

"Royal Rife" at website soul-guidance.com

"Examination under the Rife microscope of specimens ... leaves no doubt of the accurate visualization of objects or particulate matter by direct observation at the extremely high magnification ... obtained with this instrument."

Dr. Edward C. Rosenow in *Science* magazine, August 26, 1932

(Dr. Rosenow was head of experimental bacteriology at the Mayo Foundation from 1915 to 1944. *Science* magazine has long been the most prominent science journal in the USA. Rosenow declared to the "science community" that he saw magnification of about 8000X in Rife's #2 microscope. When the best optical microscope of the time obtained about 2000-2500X magnification. What Rosenow was stating for the scientific record in August 1932 in *Science* was that a history-making advance for science had occurred! The #3 Rife microscope or "Universal" was not built until 1933, and first displayed in San Diego in August and September 1933. Yet naysayers continue to claim that no one in the "peer-reviewed" science literature ever saw superior magnification and resolution in any Rife microscope! Such critics are lying as Rosenow's words prove.)

"Peering deeper into the microbiology milieu than anyone had ever done before, Rife clearly ... was able to see his specimens in vivo. In watching life processes under unprecedented magnification, Rife accomplished a feat that has not been reproduced by orthodox science nearly a century later."

The Medical Racket (2014) by Wade Frazier

"The key here is that Rife knew the resonant frequency of the virus ... in question. The specific rate of vibration was charted and cataloqued. Using a simple principle of physics, Rife understood that if he overloaded the cell with the same frequencies, it would eventually disintegrate ... replicate Rife's work ... so that the resonant frequencies of various diseases could be cataloqued and hopefully cured. The cost is minimal, the benefit to humankind -- incalculable."

Transcending the Speed of Light (2008)
by Mark Seifer, Ph.D. (Seifer is author of
Wizard: The Life and Times of Nikola Tesla)

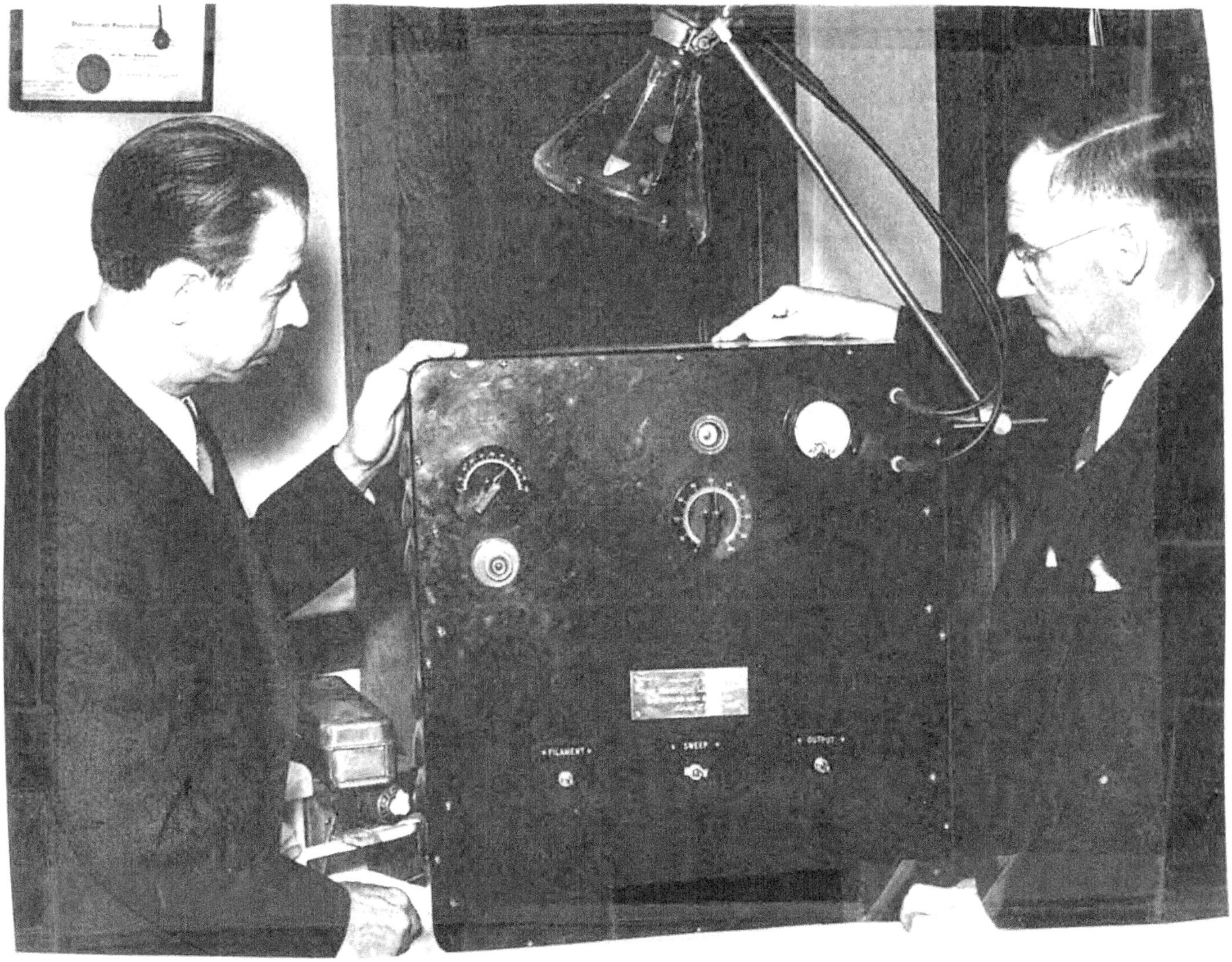

Royal Rife (left) with his engineer Philip Hoyland (right) in 1938. They are showing the Beam Ray company's prize frequency instrument, the #5 or Beam Ray Clinical instrument. This prototype had enormous success in healing microbe-caused diseases. Modern "Rife" frequency devices are derived from this model, are attempts to improve on it, or are rip-off forgeries.

"Discovery that disease organisms, including one occurring in dread cancer, can be killed by bombarding them with radio waves tuned to a particular length for each kind of organism, was claimed today by a San Diego scientist, Royal R. Rife ... Rife commented ...'these waves, or this ray, as the frequencies might be called, have been shown to possess the power of devitalizing disease organisms, of killing them, when tuned to an exact wave length, or frequency.' "

"Dread Disease Germs Destroyed by Rays: Cancer Blow Seen After 18 Year Toil" by Newell Jones. *San Diego Evening Tribune*, May 6, 1938.

"Rife was a master toolmaker and he knew a tremendous amount about optics. And he was also a visionary in his approach. He thought outside the box; he drew outside the lines. And this is why he created something that no one has duplicated since then."

Michael Coyle, Ph.D., Microscopy, from video, "The Rise and Fall of a Scientific Genius" by Sean Montgomery.

"The future of medicine is in light and electromagnetic fields. Once we find a way of manipulating and controlling electromagnetic fields, we will be able to cure just about any disease ... Probably the guy who knew the most was Royal R. Rife."

Evaluating Alternative Cancer Therapies (1998)
by David J. Hess, Ph.D. Rutgers University Press

"A 'rush order' for one of the 'universal microscopes' might be filled in two years, Rife's aide explained. A year or more would be required to make the blueprints alone ... They would cost about a quarter of a million dollars each. Alice in Wonderland had less to amaze her than a stranger to the Rife lab. Rife has recorded on film the life span of many germs. Associated with Rife is a corps of scientists and experts in the radio, physics and medical fields."

"San Diego Microscope Magnifies 30,000 Times"
by Gene Steck, *San Diego Union* May 8, 1938

"The greatest advance in medical science since Pasteur discovered disease germs ... the new polarized light, quartz microscope of Dr. Royal Rife of San Diego ... ten times more powerful than any microscope ever built." Los Angeles Evening Express, December 3, 1933.)

"The micro-photos published in the 1944 Smithsonian Report are indisputably beyond the capability of any resolution that was available at the time, and they have been confirmed by electron microscope since then ... the instrument that produced this was able to produce a resolution which we were not able to obtain except with the electron microscope many years later. This has resolution down in the neighborhood of about 20 angstroms, at least, and nobody had been able to do that. All you have to do is the arithmetic, the object size, the size of the specimen times the magnification, is equal to the image size ... We can compare the distance and we get a ratio, which is exactly comparable to what we know from modern electron microscopy."

John Hubbard, M.D., Ph.D.
Professor of Pathology
State University of New York, Buffalo

(This quotation is from "Great Revolutionary Leader of Alternative Medicine" by Richard C. Niemtzou, M.D., Ph.D., M.P.H., *The Journal of Alternative and Complementary Medicine*, August 2002, pages 688-702, at liebertpub.com.)

"Hubbard recognized the extraordinary features of the pictures, the uncanny resolution of detail, the fantastic magnification values (one order higher than standard optical scopes), the clear imaging of certain structural features within the specimens (the existence of which had previously only been suspected by microbiologists -- never seen and confirmed.) Here it was, the ultimate microscope. A tool that could open the still-murky world of germs and spill all the remaining secrets out onto the table. A tool that could help answer just about any question that a microbiologist could ask."

"Requiem for Royal Rife" by Shawn Montgomery
lifetechnologynewsblogspot.com

"To block his growing network of clinicians and researchers, the medical profession persuaded a disgruntled partner of Rife to sue the company, and it threatened loss of license to doctors who used the therapy ... as a result of the trial, Rife ended up an alcoholic and nearly bankrupt, and subseqently the clinics were closed."

"Suppression, Bias and Selection in Science"
by David J. Hess, Ph.D.
Accountability in Research, Vol. 6

"The scientist is Dr. Royal Rife ... who recently built the microscope and thereby attracted the attention of scientists all over the world ... Variable beams of monochromatic (one color) light are bent at an angle of incidence corresponding to and coordinated with the vibratory rate of the organism being examined. In this manner the minute granule ... is 'stained.' "

"Self-trained S. D. Scientist Builds Famous Microscope; Dr. Royal Rife Attracts Attention of Colleagues World Over With Instrument"
by L. E. Claypool *San Diego Union* April 16, 1934

"The implications were profound. He had seemingly found a way to selectively destroy ... pathogens without damaging a human cell."

"The End to all Disease"
Everyday Practical Electronics March 2001
(British Mass Market Magazine)

"This represented a major medical discovery of greatest value to all humanity ... The world potential of this system was staggering."

Lost Science by Gerry Vassilatos

"... a San Diego biologist was developing a microscope that today stands as one of biology's greatest breakthroughs. Royal Rife ... stands among science's giants."

The Medical Racket by Wade Frazier

"Let us hope that the work of Rife will be resurrected and that a substantial investment will be made in progressing this important area of medical research to the benefit of everyone. Unfortunately, for too long powerful organizations with vested interests have suppressed development and research in this area." (Underlining added.)

"The End to all Disease"
Everyday Practical Electronics *March 2001*
(British mass market magazine)

"There are a number of alternative healing therapies that work so well and cost so little ... that Organized Medicine, the Food and Drug Administration, and their overlords in the Pharmaceutical Industry (The Big Three) would rather the public not know about them. The reason is obvious. The Big Three have collectively engaged in a medical conspiracy ... to promote the use of drug medicine while simultaneously creating restrictive, controlling mechanisms ... designed to limit and stifle ... non-drug, alternative modalities.

"Royal Rife ... was able to destroy all manner of disease organisms (including cancer organisms) by merely tuning the generator to the correct resonant frequency of these organisms." (Underlining added.)

"Forbidden Cures" by Ken Adachi at aurimedia.net

"10,000 Americans die of cancer every week while your agency took more than 3 months to reply to my very serious interest in the potential of this Rife cancer therapy. This suggests a fundamental error in FDA's understanding of its obligations and accountability to the American people and America's guiding principles.

"There appears to be serious, factual errors in FDA's published statements concerning Rife's work. This, added to the 3 plus months to organize your reply is not entirely acceptable. Could someone attempt to answer my inquiry?" (Underlining added.)

Letter to FDA Commissioner Jane E. Henney, June 27, 2000 from
U.S. Congressman Cliff Stearns, Health & Environment Subcommittee

"Royal Raymond Rife of San Diego invented a high magnification, high-resolution light microscope. This meant that he could see unstained living cells, unlike the dead specimens seen under an electron microscope. Basically, he developed an electromagnetic frequency generator which he could tune to the natural frequency of the micro-organism under study. Further, he learned that certain frequencies could kill specific bacterial forms.

"New discoveries in biophysics not only shed light on the illumination process of Rife's microscope, they explain how he could selectively explode viruses. His concept of shape-changing bacteria indicate that traditional germ theory is incomplete. Despite documented cures, his non-drug, electrical treatment of diseases was not welcomed by a powerful medical union."

"Top Ten Impossible Inventions That Work"
by Jeanne Manning at website MERLib.org
(Modern Energy Research Library)

"Rife repeated his experiments with thousands of samples and reproduced the same effect every time ... he was unable to find any frequency that would cause human ... tissue cells to explode in the same way -- meaning that the technique could selectively destroy bacteria and other pathogens in the human body without destroying human cells! The implications were profound. Rife had found a way to selectively destroy invading bacteria and other pathogens in the human body without causing damage in any human cells."

"Electromedicine Modalities"
September 7, 2017
samedaypapers.com

"Royal Rife's discovery of the frequency characteristics of organisms led him to believe that each individual type of microorganism should have a resonant frequency that would be detrimental to it. He believed that if such a frequency could be found and applied, the rays would be fatal to the disease organism but not to the normal cells that didn't vibrate at the frequency being sent into the patient. This proved to be exactly right."

"The Rife Microscope and Generator"
by Dennis Myers, M.D.
members.limetro.com.au

"Rife frequency therapy, put simply, is a term for the use of ultrasound to kill germs ... Most every germ or pathogen has its own resonant frequency at which it will vibrate and shake until its structure is disrupted ... Once the basic principles of this science are grasped, it is quite easy to see how this really works and how it can be applied to all manner of pathogen-based diseases.

"The applications of this are so wide and so effective that even in Rife's day, the orthodox authorities such as the FDA and the AMA fought hard and long to keep this science away from the public's awareness."

"Rife Therapy and Treatment Explained'
by casperdude
Alternativemedicinetruth.blogspot.ca

"Dr. Royal Rife (1888-1971) was a brilliant, passionate scientist who discovered that every virus, bacterium, parasite and pathogen is sensitive to a special frequency of sound and can be destroyed by intensifying that frequency until it literally explodes, much like an intense musical note can shatter a crystal wine glass. He called this the mortal oscillatory rate (MOR).

"We are in a period of dramatic change in the healthcare system. Energy medicine has a huge role to play in this process. The reason is that conventional Western medicine is the only medical system in world history that has virtually ignored energetics. Energetic concepts are part of nearly all of the complementary and alternative therapies that the public is enthusiastically moving towards."

Energy Medicine: The Scientific Basis (2016)
by James Oschman, Ph.D.

"The Rife Raytube Therapy was the only time in history that viruses could be selectively and dramatically destroyed ... Dr. Rife had developed and implemented what no contemporary medical research group had ever conceived."

Lost Science
by Gerry Vasilatos

"A recent breakthrough in high-intensity focused ultrasound (HIFU) technology has proved its use as an effective cancer treatment ... The findings were published in the Journal of Applied Physics.

"As one might imagine ... I couldn't help but think of the medical industry's assault on Royal Rife ... he claimed to have experimented using different sound waves to find the right frequency for various viruses which he claimed caused sarcomas and carcinomas. Until, that is, he was shut down.

"If there's a lesson here, it's that this idea has been around for a very long time, and ... Dr. Rife's ideas were essentially confirmed. That also means a cure or technique was suppressed for almost eighty years, while big pharma and big medicine cut, hacked, sawed, radiated, and chemo-ed people with cures almost as bad as the diseases." (Underlining added.)

"Sound Versus Cancer? Shades of Royal Rife" by Joseph P. Farrell
gizedeathstar.com September 21, 2018

"The organisms Rife was trying to observe were too small to absorb existing acid or aniline dye stains, which in any case killed the organisms. Instead, he experimented with light frequencies, and found that each type of microbe could be made to fluoresce using a resonant frequency. He redesigned the microscope to incorporate these light-staining capabilities.

"This enabled him to forego the use of chemical dyes and observe life on the microbial level without killing it. Rife became not only the first man to observe life forms at the ultra-microscope level, but to observe them alive, to watch them live.

"By extension of the light-staining techniques, he discovered that specific frrequencies could be used to destroy micro-organisms. Hit the right frequency and they just popped. He called it the Mortal Oscillatory Rate, and he began the painstaking work of logging the MORS of some fifty types of pathogens.

"From the legacy of Tesla, our understanding reaches out into the cosmos. With Rife, it goes within and deep into the microcosmos."

"The Microscopist" by Paul Dunbar
thelethaltext.me April 24, 2018

"Rife may be the most promising and unknown therapy in modern times. It was so effective that it was suppressed with a force and a vengeance that even drove it from the history books."

"Alternatives To Surgery and Drugs"
by John Q. Citizen
ahm – portal.com/Alternatives (2015)

"In the 1930's and 1940's, Royal Raymond Rife revolutionized everything that has been done before or since in high-resolution optical microscopy. He also revolutionized everything before or since in cellular biology. He carried cellular structure far beyond anything ever dreamed of in his time or previously.

"With his Universal Microscope, Rife ... could examine living viruses, living bacteria, and other as-yet-undiscovered living organisms and living energy forms that no other microscope before or since could see. In one swoop medical science could have jumped a century ahead. The ruthlesss suppression of Rife and his scientific breakthrough was one of the most dastardly deeds ever perpetrated by the orthodox scientific establishment.

"Rife's revolutionary work ... incurred the unending, total opposition of powerful individuals controlling the direction of biology and medical science for their own personal gain.

"Rife was hounded into court on trumped up charges ... he emerged a shaken, broken man and an alcoholic. His work was suppressed ... He died without ever being vindicated for his marvelous, world-shaking discoveries."

Extraordinary Biology (Chapter Five)
by Tom Bearden
website cheniere.org

"What happened to Rife ... It was what happened when medicine was a monopoly. The goal of any monopoly is to gain market share while destroying all competition."

David Bonello
November 30, 2017
wellnessjourney.org

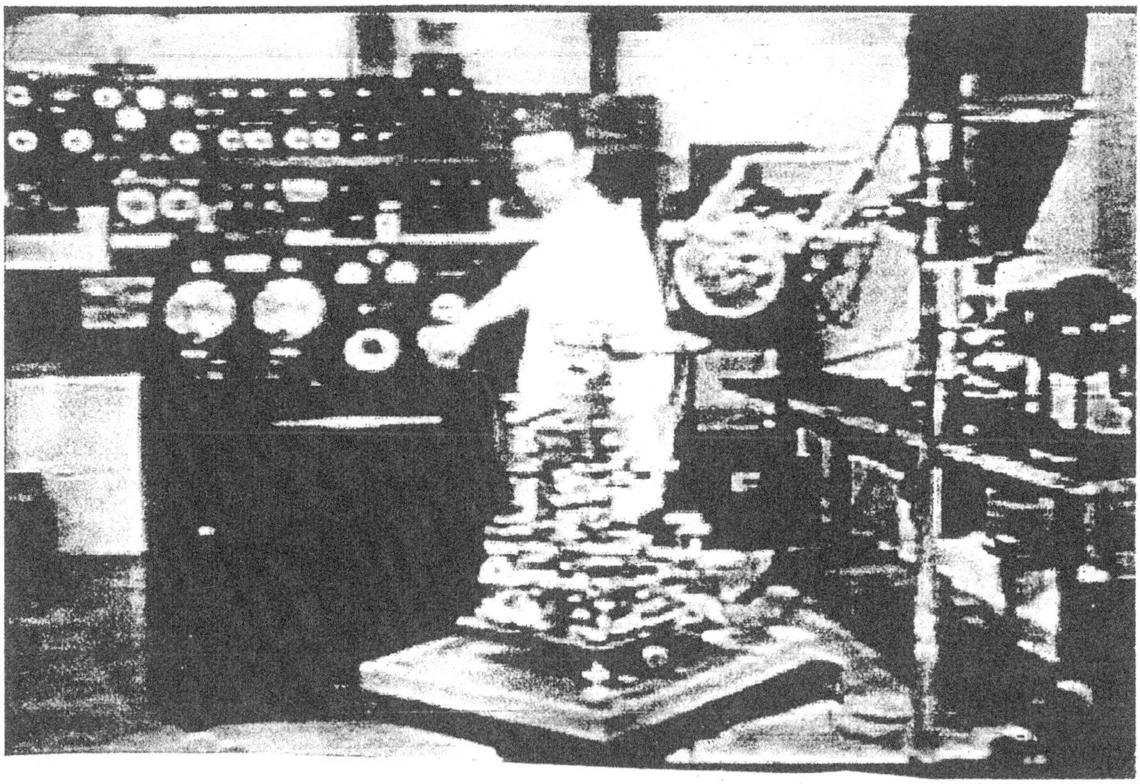

Royal Rife in his laboratory. The Universal Microscope is in front of him. Above and to the right of the microscope is a glass bulb where a flash appears when frequencies are sent out. The "correct" frequency immediately kills the microbe that is being studied in a slide under the microscope. Rife spent up to 48 hours at a time watching one frequency after another being tested against a specific microbe to determine which would kill the cause of a given disease! What Rife termed its "M.O.R." -- Mortal Oscillatory Rate.

As Rife's associate Ben Cullen recalled, "I've seen Roy sit in that doggone seat without moving, watching the changes in the frequency, watching when the time would come when the virus in the slide would be destroyed. Twenty-four hours was nothing for him. Forty-eight hours. He had done it many times. Sit there without moving. He wouldn't touch anything except a little water. His nerves were just like cold steel. He never moved. His hands never quivered."

" Of course he would train beforehand and go through a very careful workout afterward to build himself up again. But that is what I would call one of the most magnificent sights of human control and endurance I've ever seen."

"I made a steady pilgrimage to Rife's garage where we set up a shop with machinery to build his microscopes ... Rife's third microscope, the big Universal Microscope ... he ground many of his own lenses. He developed a system of grinding his own lenses and I watched him do it. He mounted them, of course, in this 21-bend microscope which is the Universal ... he actually had figured out the parabolas and then ground the lenses to those parabolas ... he had prisms located at each corner of the bend from one side to the other and they (were) interposed between those lenses, because the prisms themselves did not magnify ... simply they carried the image from one magnification to another on up through the objectives lens to the oculars ... He always interposed a lens between two prisms at each end." (Underlining added.)

"Interview With Ben Cullen by John Hubbard"
from "Requiem For Royal Rife" by Shawn Montgomery

"Another feature was the microscope's extraordinary resolution, its ability to reveal the most minute of component parts of any specimen so that each may be seen distinctly and separately from the others. Imagine two extremely thin parallel lines. When they can be clearly distinguished you are still within the microscope's range of resolution. If the parallel lines blur together, high magnification will only enlarge the distortion and limit of resolution has been reached. With a resolving power of 31,000 diameters -- as against 2,000 to 2,500 for the laboratory microscopes in common use in that day ... Rife's devices could focus clearly on five lines of a standardized grid, whereas an ordinary microscope could do no better than examine fifty lines, and with considerable abberation." (Underlining added.)

"What Has Become of the Rife Microscope?"
by Christopher Bird, *New Age Journal* March 1976

"The Rife Universal Microscope was and remains a very sophisticated step beyond the usual understanding of light optics. The system provided reportedly 60,000X magnification with extremely high resolving power. It is capable of employing monochromatic light in order to fluoresce all strains of microorganisms individually, thereby marking them for examination and treatment." (Underlining added.)

"The Super Microscope" by Michael Coyle, Ph.D.
website dreddymd.com

Through years of dedicated research in microbiology and the invention of a radical design for optical microscopes, Rife demonstrated that ordinary sized bacteria can be reduced to a smaller "filtered form" of virus size! They are now called nanobacteria. Rife also showed that these disease-causing nanobacteria can be destroyed by a specific electronic frequency. Tuberculosis nanobacteria have a "signature" oscillatory rate. The cancer nanobacteria (BX) has a different, but unchanging "killer" frequency which has a proven capability to reverse a person's cancer condition IF their cancer was caused by the BX!!

"By resolution, we refer to the ability of the microscope to distinguish a small object. In other words, something like looking at a medical doctor's eye chart, and specifying the smallest print one can clearly see. Resolution is often referred to as resolving power.

"Much of today's knowledge of virus structure and shape comes from the use of electron microscopes. They bombard the object viewed with a fierce rain of energetic electrons. These instruments see nothing of the functioning of the virus, for they kill it instantly, to view the virus. With Rife's Universal Microscope, the dynamic living function of the virus could be observed without killing it. In addition, Rife's microscope ... revealed living halos around living organisms that other microscopes could not see." (Underlining added.)

Extraordinary Biology (Chapter Five) by Tom Bearden
website cheniere.org

"He (Rife) built a chart that was sort of like the Periodic Chart. There were even 7 or 9 families ... All the pathogens fit one or another of these columns. All the pathogens getting down below worms and so forth. Viruses, bacteria of various types, and fungi of various types, and on up through an evolutionary-type ladder ... All human pathogens fell onto this chart ... And the key to each of these columns -- which would have a very small virus at the bottom and a pretty good size fungus at the top -- that within that column was a single T-protein."

"Requiem for Royal Rife: The Hubbard Interviews"
Quoting Rife's neighbor Robert Z. Page
By Shawn Montgomery at svpwiki.com Aug 10, 2006

Part III

The 1934 Cancer Clinical Trial in La Jolla, California when Royal Rife's Frequency Therapy was tested and successfully cured 16 "hopeless" patients.

"Every third day, each patient sat a few feet from the ray machine for 3 minutes. Spacing of the treatments 'devitalized' the cancer one tissue layer at a time. It also allowed the body to heal and rid itself of toxins. Within 3 months, 14 of the 16 cancer patients had recovered. The other 2 had clean bills of health within the next 6 weeks.

"On May 6, 1938, the *San Diego Evening Tribune* announced that after 18 years of trial and error in his Point Loma lab, Rife had isolated a cancer organism and a means of arresting it. He compared the ray to compatible tuning forks. When one vibrates, sound waves cause the other to vibrate as well." (Underlining added.)

"Royal Raymond Rife: Into The Micro Beyond"
by Jeff Smith at *San Diego Reader* February 12, 2012

"You can imagine what they gave us. They came in ambulances twice a week ... photographs before and after. This board -- six of the most outstanding medical men of the United States ... Our board pronounced them (patients) clinically cured."

History of a Successful Cure for Cancer (1953)
by Royal R. Rife (at National Library of Medicine)

Part III. The 1934 Cancer Clinical Trial In La Jolla, California

The 1934 Cancer Clinical Trial in La Jolla, California successfully cured 16 of 16 terminal cancer and tuberculosis patients. It was sponsored by the University of Southern California to test Royal Rife's Frequency Destruction of the BX nanobacteria which Rife isolated from human cancer. The following persons were the primary doctors, academic witnesses, or observers:

Dr. Milbank Johnson, Professor of Physiology and Clinical Medicine at U.S.C. headed the clinical trial. Other physicians included Whalen Morrison Chief Surgeon of the Santa Fe Railway, George C. Dock, M.D., internationally famous, George C. Fischer, M.D., Children's Hospital in New York, Arthur I. Kendall, Dept of Bacteriology, Northwestern University, (America's "Pasteur"), Dr. Zite, M.D., professor of pathology at Chicago University, Rufas B. Von KleinSchmidt, President of the University of Southern California, Dr. Carl Meyer, Ph.D, head of the Department of Bacteriological Research at the Hooper Foundation in San Francisco, Dr. Kopps, M.D., of the Metabolic Clinic in La Jolla, California, Alvin Foord, M.D. and pathologist for the trial, and Dr. James Couche, M.D. of San Diego.

In 1956, 22 years after the trial, Dr. James Couche made the following declaration:

"I would like to make this historical record of the amazing scientific wonders regarding the efficacy of the frequencies of the Royal R. Rife Frequency Instrument.

"When I was told about Dr. Rife and his frequency instrument at the Ellen Scripps home near the Scripps Institute Annex some twenty-two years ago, I went out to see about it and became very interested in the cases which he had there. And the thing that brought me into it more quickly than anything was a man who had a cancer of the stomach. Rife was associated at that time with Dr. Milbank Johnson, M.D. who was then president of the Medical Association of Los Angeles, a very wealthy man and a very big man in the medical world -- the biggest in Los Angeles and he had hired this annex for this demonstration over a summer of time.

"In that period of time I saw many things and the one that impressed me the most was a man who staggered onto a table, just on the last end of cancer; he was a bag of bones. As he lay on the table, Dr. Rife and Dr. Johnson said, 'Just feel that man's stomach.' So I put my hand on the cavity where his stomach was underneath and it was just a cavity almost, because he was so thin; his backbone and his belly were just about touching each other.

"I put my hand on his stomach which was just one solid mass, just about what I could cover with my hand, somewhat like the shape of a heart. It was absolutely solid! And I thought to myself, well, nothing can be done for that. However, they gave him a treatment with the Rife frequencies and in the course of time over a period of six weeks to two months, to my astonishment, he completely recovered. He got so well that he asked permission to go to El Centro as he had a farm there and he wanted to see about his stock. Dr. Rife said, 'Now you haven't the strength to drive to El Centro.'

" 'Oh yes,' said he. 'I have, but I'll have a man to drive me there.' As a matter of fact, the patient drove his own car there and when he got down to El Centro he had a sick cow and he stayed up all night with it. The next day he drove back without any rest whatsoever -- so you can imagine how he had recovered.

"I saw other cases that were very interesting. Then I wanted a copy of the frequency instrument. I finally bought one of these frequency instruments and established it in my office.

"I saw some very remarkable things resulting from it in the course of over twenty years."

In 1953 when Rife finished his book, he wrote this about the 1934 cancer clinical trial"

"With the frequency instrument treatment, no tissue is destroyed, no pain is felt, no noise is audible, and no sensation is noticed. A tube lights up and three minutes later the treatment is completed. The virus or bacteria is destroyed and the body then recovers itself naturally from the toxic effect of the virus or bacteria. Several diseases may be treated simultaneosly.

"The first clinical work on cancer was completed under the supervision of Milbank Johnson, M.D. which was set up under a Special Medical Research Committee of the University of Southern California. 16 cases were treated at the clinic for many types of malignancy. After 3 months, 14 of those so-called hopeless cases were signed off as clinically cured by the staff of five medical doctors and Dr. Alvin G. Foord, Pathologist. The treatments consisted of 3 minutes duration using the frequency instrument which was set at the mortal oscillatory rate for 'BX' or cancer (at 3 day intervals). It was found that the elapsed time between treatments attains better results than the cases treated daily. This gives the lymphatic system an opportunity to absorb and cast off the toxic condition which is produced by the devitalized particles of the 'BX' virus."

Date: December 1, 1953 Written by Royal R. Rife

Three years after the successful USC clinical success, an 82-year-old man from Chicago with an awful facial cancer became a patient of Dr. Richard Hamer in San Diego, California. Dr. Hamer had a Rife frequency instrument and was curing many patients of different maladies. He hired two operators and was treating 40 patients a day. This excerpt is from a longer taped interview of Ben Cullen, titled "Ben Cullen Talks About Dr. Rife May 7, 1960" at rifevideos.com. (Underlining Added.)

"The condition was a ... cancer which started on one side of his face, took in his eyelid, ate the eyelid off, this lobe of the ear, and around here, down around this side and finally into the right atrium basin ... Dr. Hamer said he didn't see any reason why this particular type of cancer wouldn't react to the Rife Ray.

"So the gentleman began to fly back and forth three times a week. Then he saw the improvement and he took residence here for six months. At the end of six months, this gentleman had one little black spot right here in the area, which was just simply a little scab which Dr. Hamer said would tumble off in a few days, or a week. So he went back to Chicago. And when he got back there he just couldn't keep still. He couldn't keep quiet and he talked to everyone about this marvelous healing. Those who knew him from before ... were utterly amazed because he had nice, new, smooth skin just like a baby's.

"So this gentleman in Chicago talked about the cancer healing. Fishbein of the American Medical Association ... heard about this man ... He got from him the story of this Rife Ray treatment. And Fishbein made every effort to ... buy into the corporation that was manufacturing these machines. The machines were manufactured in San Diego. It was a California corporation and it was a closed one. There was no stock for sale. Two men from Los Angeles came down here. We again said we were not prepared to enlarge our activity.

"That was too much for Fishbein. So he requested that some effort be made to find a weak spot in our organization. Which he did ... in one of the members of our board of directors (Philip Hoyland, Rife's engineer). And that man was paid a nice fee ($10,000) if he would precipitate some sort of condition which would make it possible for the company to be thrown into receivership. This was done and in due course of time, the case was sent to be tried in Judge Kelly's court in San Diego. The case took a year and three days to prosecute ... Kelly gave the corporation a clean bill of health. One of the members of the corporation was completely broke and so was the corporation.

"In addition to that, the American Medical Association had sent out word that the doctors who were found operating the Rife Ray Machine, two weeks from the receipt of the notice, would lose their membership in the AMA. The doctors were compelled to rid their offices of these machines. The company manufacturing these machines folded."

"Dr. Morris Fishbein (1889-1976) ... became head of the AMA, a position he used to enrich himself and crush legitimate therapies out of existence ... As head of the AMA, he decided which drugs could be sold to the public based only on how much advertising money he could extract from drug manufacturers ... It was irrelevant if the drugs worked. Fishbein was a shakedown artist.

"The worst of Fishbein's sins was his destruction of Royal Rife ... The trial of 1939 put an end to the proper scientific investigation of Rife's frequency machine ... We are 80 years behind where we should be because of one despicable man, Morris Fishbein, who used the State to halt the advance of medicine, and to line his own pockets."

"Morris Fishbein -- AMA Enemy of American Health"
by Bob Wallace at LewRockwell.com

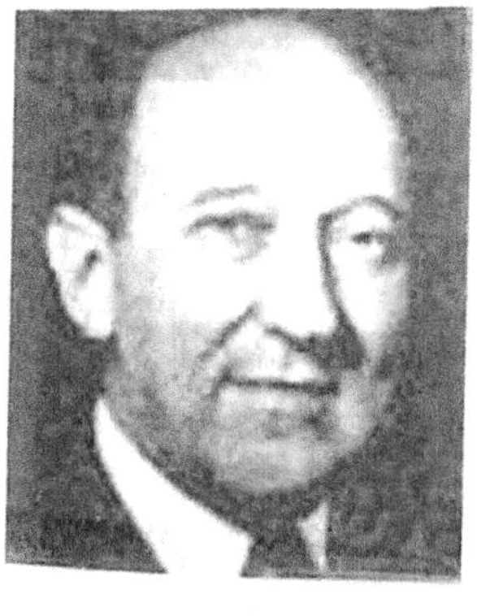

Morris Fishbein

The Modern Cancer Treatment Industry

"... chemotherapy and radiotherapy, the two cornerstones of modern orthodox cancer treatment are not effective treatments to the vast majority of cancer patients, and yet these 'treatments' are given protected monopathy status by most developed countries around the world, effectively sentencing 96%-98% of cancer sufferers to hugely destructive and painful treatments ...

"So going back to cancer treatment, we see an insanely conventional cancer treatment industry ineffective for the vast majority of cancer sufferers and based mostly on spurious science, but one that has been granted a monopoly by our governments to prevent other treatments ... from even being discussed ... The situation cannot be in the public interest ... the whole edifice of modern cancer care is rotten at the core because policy is controlled by big business." (Underlining added.)

"Cancer Treatment Protection Racket" by John Smith energygrid.com

"... there is massive deception and manipulation ... to keep us from investigating low profitable treatment that could upset the multi-billion-dollar plans and ploys of the drug industry ... we will never reach that ... 'world without cancer' unless we root out the corruption that has overtaken most of the leadership of the oncology profession." (Underlining added.)

Ralph Moss, Ph.D., "Cancer Inside Story" lifeextension.com May 2022

Dr. Moss: "... we should imitate and copy the laws in Germany that they put in place for accessing these treatments. There is an attitude of respect for the individual and treating people as adults ... Responsible people who are not going to abuse the system. And it works for them. This has been since the 1970s. They've had this legal structure. They established commissions to study the different kinds of treatment. But basically what we would call naturopathic treatment was put on an equal footing with allopathic treatment. I've never seen a doctor punished or 'persecuted' in the 25 years since I've been going to Germany." (Underlining added.)

"Dr. Ralph Moss Interview" by Chris Wark chrisbeatcancer.com (2020)

Why We Have Todays' Cancer HORRORS

There was something about the AMA's boss Morris Fishbein's crime that only listing the bare facts of his attempt to steal Rife's marvelous therapy, and failing that, his suppression of its further medical use, fails to convey the enormity of Fishbein's evil act. Perhaps only the following description expresses some accurate feeling of the tragedy wrought by Fishbein's foul deed:

"Morris Fishbein. The single dominant force in the AMA at that time, he was belligerent, ruthless and it is to be noted that he never practiced medicine as an MD for even a single day in his life past his residency. He was a smothering and potent personality, revealing him as a political animal of the first order.

"Fishbein sent a fateful message ... seeking to buy into Rife's work and his new company, Beam Ray. Rife refused. This was the start of the end. When the devil knocks there is little choice but to let him in, lest he burn the house to the ground.

"Rife was a patient, genteel and kind man, an intellectual, engineer and scientist who was about to enter an ugly bully's world of money, brutal assault, cruelty and blatant injustice: the American legal system. Cancer he had cured, but politics? This would soon metastasize and consume him.. The opposing lawyer cut into him and attacked him. Rife was unprepared and although his case was settled in due course in Rife's favor, the experience destroyed him on the human level ... his nerves gave way ... Thus began his deterioration into alcoholism and depression. Beam Ray would be ruined, Rife shattered and the cure for cancer snuffed out. What Fishbein could not own, he would destroy.

"Was there a cover up? Do examine the video presentation of Rife's laboratory. Observe the massive investment and many pieces of advanced equipment Rife created. Observe the highly advanced work and surgical techniques. Was there a cover up? Ask yourself. What happened to all this? It appears to have vanished without a trace. Cancer has been cured since 1934, and no one knows it." (Underlining added.)

Excerpted from a longer piece titled, "An Open Letter Regarding Cancer" by Richard Lawrence Norman, Editor in chief, *Mind* magazine at website editor@journalofunconsciouspsychology.com, and by Jeremy Dunning-Davies, Department of Mathematics and Physics (retired), University of Hull, England, and Institute of Basic Research, Palm Harbor, Florida, at website j.dunning-davies@hull.ac.uk.

AMA Shakedown Artist
The Man Who Corrupted Medicine

"Oncologist Azra Raza of Columbia University Medical School ... 'There is a crisis in oncology. Cost of cancer care will consume more than 80% of cancer spending by 2030 . Only 6% of cancer drugs approved between 2006 - 2017 showed meaningful, measurable quality of life improvement while a good 70% showed 0% improvement in survival. Twenty years after the human genome was sequenced and despite an overwhelming focus on gene-centric research, very little has changed for the cancer patient ... The same slash-poison-burn. And the outcome for the 30% we are not curing ... is no different in 2021 than it was in 1930.' " (Underlining added.)

"The First Cell" by John Hewitt
website medicalpress.com May 2021

Yet official medicine refuses to test Rife's resonance therapy! The blackout that began with AMA boss Morris Fishbein continues. The American Cancer Society still tells lies about "Rife being disproved." The National Cancer Instiute (NCI) remains opposed to fair, independent trials involving modern frequency instruments that have cured some patients of cancer! Cancer researchers live in a Pharma world where they never learn anything about Royal Rife's microscope or the use of resonance to destroy the BX cause of some cancers! This is corrupt "medical politics" which suppresses a breakthrough Biophysics therapy!

This Galileo-like blacklisting of revolutionary science ideas needs exposure and condemnation so future "controversial" breakthroughs have safeguarding.

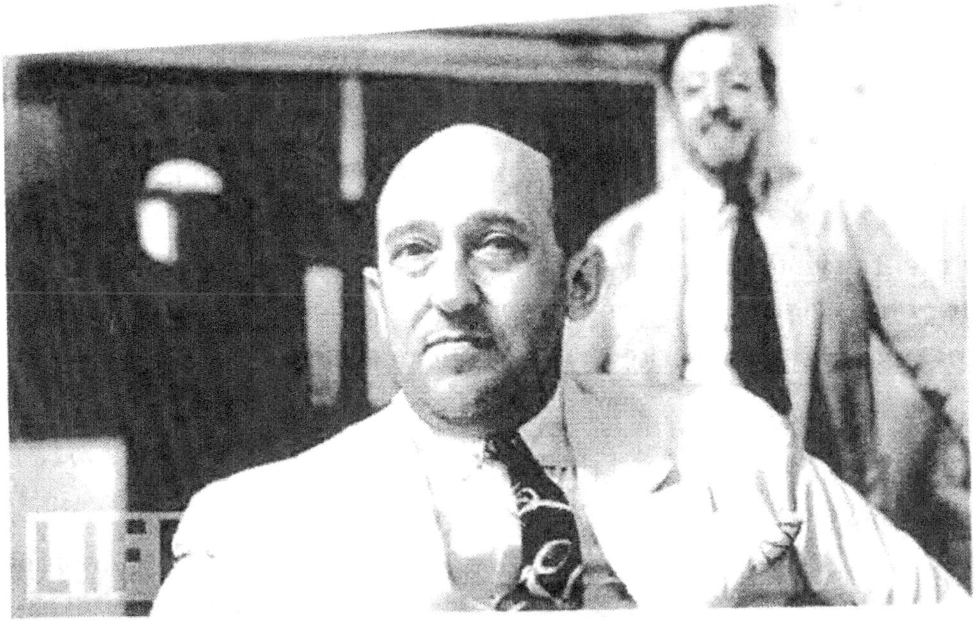

Morris Fishbein

"The isolation (discovery) of cancer virus and other micro-organisms was an accomplishment with which I felt a great deal of pride. Finally, in 1931, I discovered the ... cancer virus and the successful treatment for cancer and other diseases by actual observation of (through) the ... microscope while applying the frequency instrument ... With the frequency instrument, no tissue is destroyed, no pain is felt, no noise is audible, and no sensation is noticed. A tube lights up and 3 minutes later the treatment is completed. The virus or bacteria is destroyed and the body then recovers itself naturally from the toxic effect of the virus and bacteria."

History of the Development of a
Successful Treatment for Cancer (1953) by Royal Rife

"The Rife BX/BY 'virus' was probably not a virus but a filterable, polymorphic, cell-wall deficient bacterium like Bacillus licheniformis ... In this regard, it appears similar to the Gregory cancer 'virus' which duplicates by cell replication, clearly not a virus. Both of these organisms are found in every cancer patient.

"Virtually all people with cancer are infected with bacillus licheniformis. The first step in dealing with cancer electronically must be to eliminate all bacillus licehniformis from the body as it appears to be both a tumor promoter and a mutagen. Tumors will tend to grow or recur with this organism present.

"Many researchers have not seen the note in Lancet, one of the leading medical journals, where scientists claimed to have sequenced the 'cancer germ.' What appears to be the Rife 'filterable bacteria' was isolated and DNA sequenced by the British researchers. Bacillus licheniformis is a pleomorphic organism that appears as rods, cocci, and fungus-like forms.

"In my view, scanning and eliminating this bacterium in the general population could reduce the incidence of cancer and improve the survival of cancer patients by 50%. This is based on my own research and that of hundreds of investigators trying to replicate Rife's early work on successful treatment of cancer patients with electronic devices."

"Rife Cancer Virus May Be
Bacillus Licheniformis" (June 15, 2017)
by Jeff Sutherland AT frequencyfoundation.com

"I have a Ph.D. in this area, 11 years on the faculty of the University of Colorado Medical School funded by the National Cancer Institute, much published research, and am still the last time I checked, one of only 300 scientists in the U.S. authorized to lead grants funded by NCI.

"Frequency therapy, properly applied, may well replace every other modality. Frequency devices can change the medical paradigm as we know it. But unfortunately, there is considerable resistance to electro-medicine.

"Healthcare is a government regulated monopoly that systematically suppresses new innovation ... powerful institutional forces fight simpler alternatives to expensive care because those alternatives threaten their livelihoods ... large amounts of money are involved." (Underlining added.)

Dr. Jeff Sutherland, Preface to
The Rife Handbook by Nenah Sylver, Ph.D.

"Healthy cells, according to Nobel Prize winner Otto Warburg, have cell voltages of 70 to 90 millivolts ... If the electrical charge of a cell drops to 50, a person has chronic fatigue and gets sick often. If the voltage drops to 15, the cell becomes cancerous. The fastest way to raise cell voltage is with a device called a MultiWave Oscillator (MWO). George Lakhovsky invented MWOs in the early 1900s.

"15 years later, Royal Rife, the inventor of the Rife machine, had an idea. If all cells have a frequency that they can be charged at, what would happen if you isolated that frequency and sent it more energy than it could handle? He surmised that just like overcharging a battery, the cell could be made to explode. Rife was right, and spent many years discovering the frequencies in which viruses and bacteria could be destroyed.

"In this sense, a Rife machine is the exact opposite of a MWO. They both rely on the same principle, that is, that life forms can absorb radio wave energy. The MWO uses that principle to strengthen the healthy cells of the body so that they can resist disease. A Rife machine uses the principle to destroy microorganisms that are causing problems ... Rife machines and MultiWave Oscillators ... two technologies from the past to help us with the diseases of the present."

"MultiWave Oscillators" by Pacific Northwest Foundation (2004)

Appendix &
Rife's Frequencies

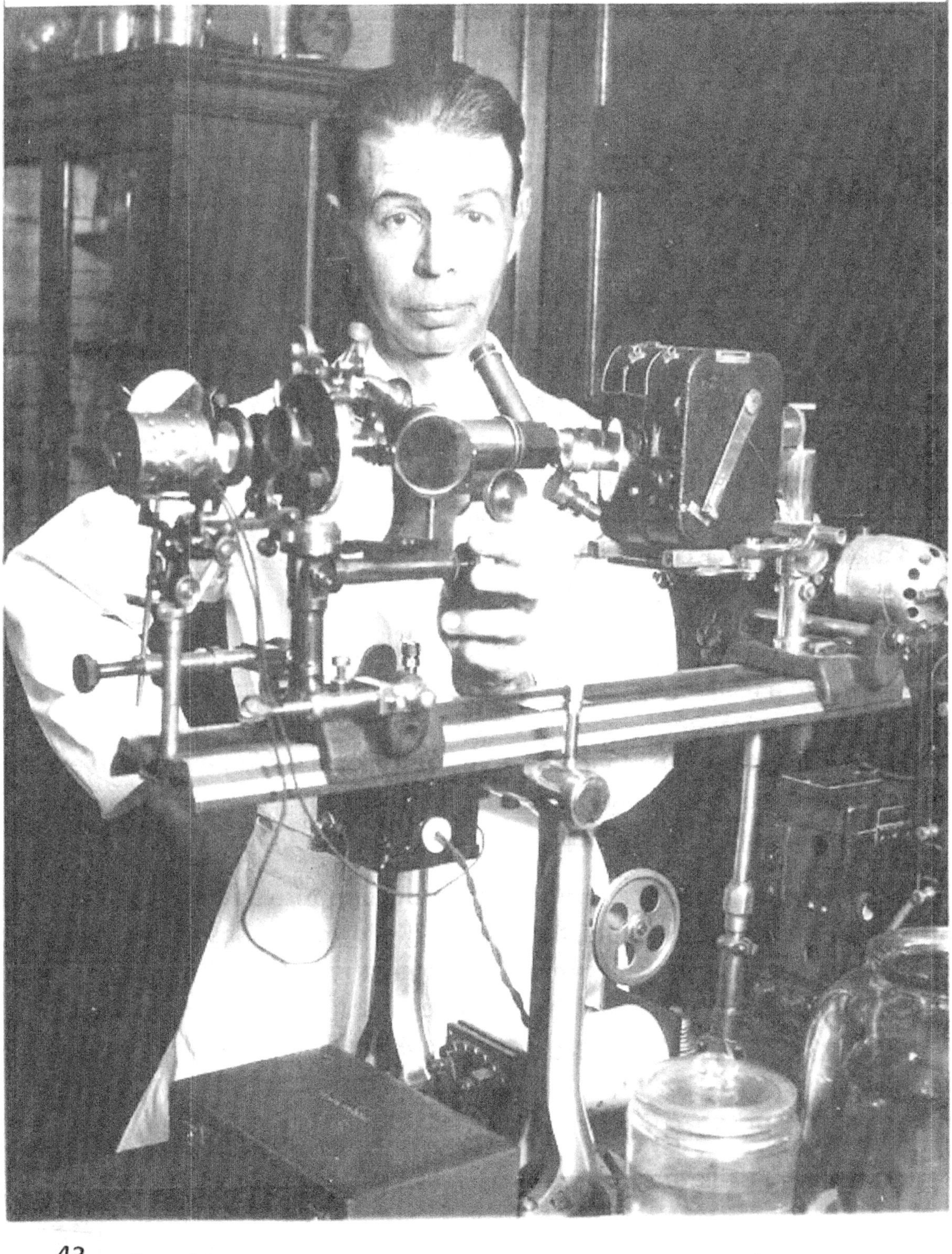

Royal Rife with one of his earliest microscope creations.

Top Scientists & Doctors Gather To Honor Royal Rife
And His Powerful New Microscope With 17,000X Magnification!

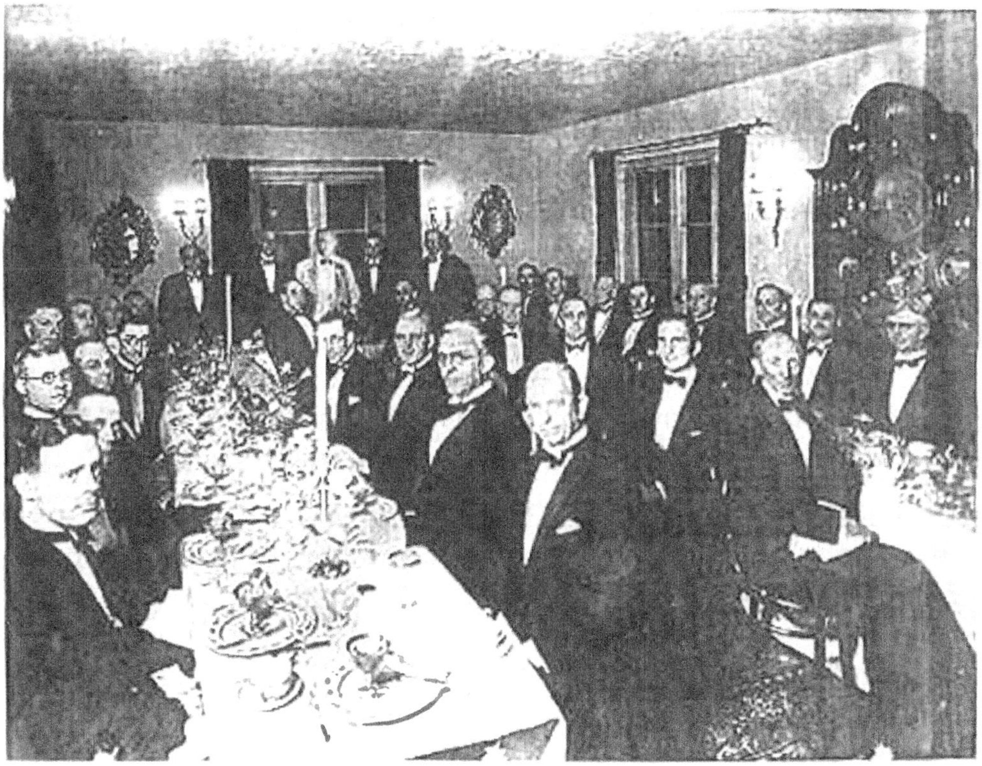

Dr. Milbank Johnson holds a dinner at his mansion in Pasadena, California to honor Royal Rife. The dinner occurred on November 20, 1931. More than 30 of the most prominent medical doctors, pathologists, and bacteriologists saw a microscope which broke the supposed magnification limits.

The Los Angeles Times of November 22, 1931 reported, "Through the use of Dr. Rife's powerful microscope, said to have a visual power of magnification to 17,000 times, compared to 2,000 of which the ordinary microscope is capable."

"Dr. Rife, by an ingenious arrangement of lenses applying an entirely new optical principle and by introducing double quartz prisms and powerful illuminating lights, has devised a microscope with a lower magnification of 5,000 times and a maximum working magnification of 17,000 times."

"Frankly dubious about the perfection of a microscope which appears to transcend the limits set by optic science, Dr. Johnson's guests expressed themselves as delighted with the visual demonstration and heartily accorded ... Dr. Rife ... a foremost place in the world's rank of scientists."

"Doctors Wait For Test Of Rife Ray"
by Newall Jones
San Diego Evening Tribune May 7 1938

"Royal Raymond Rife, San Diego scientist ... told of the latest developments made in his Pt Loma laboratory on his microscope, the first of which was announced seven years ago, and of unreported discoveries which these have made possible. Outstanding among these discoveries were the revelations of previously unseen, filter-passing, pathogenic viruses for bombardment with the Rife Ray.

" 'Physicists have always clung to the rule,' said the San Diegan, 'that any object which is smaller than one-half the wavelength of the light by which it is illuminated under the microscope cannot be seen in its true form or detail. This is true with the conventional method of optics. But these instruments introduce other methods.'

"The scientist explained the new methods and what they accomplish.

"In the standard microscope, the image of the subject being studied is projected 180 millimeters from the master lens of the objective to the eye point. By this great distance of projection, the magnification is limited.

"However, in the optical principles involved in the Rife instruments, there is virtually a tube length of 200 to 449 millimeters, but the greatest distance of projection of the image through any one media, either quartz or air, is less than 30 millimeters.

"This shortening of the distance through any one media, it was explained, allows greater magnification and eliminates chromatical, and most of the spherical aberration ... This shortening is made possible by use of quartz blocks and prisms in the body tube of the microsope to carry the vision of the image through the optical path. In the conventional microscope, the vision of the image passes through the air in the hollow tube of the instrument.

"The new instruments obtain a peak magnification of 31,000. Maximum for standard laboratory instruments is only slightly more than 1600.

"Then, in making visible the filter-passing forms of bacteria, or virus, the paramount factor of the Rife instrument is a different illuminating system, the major part of which is composed of a series of rotating, circular wedged quartz prisms. As these prisms are rotated, they increase or decrease the angle of incidence of the illuminating beam, changing the light beam frequency, or wavelength, to coordinate with the particular organism under observation."

"... quartz prisms provide the quality of light necessary to see the bacilli in color without the use of chemical stains and without injuring the organisms ... Dr. Rife ... his invention of a stabilizer for airplanes used during the World War (WWI) won him decorations from several of the allied powers."

San Diego Union December 4, 1931

"More than 75% of the organisms Rife could see with his Universal Microscope are only visible with ultra-violet light. But ultraviolet light is outside the range of human vision; it is invisible to us. Rife's brilliance allowed him to overcome this limitation by heterodyning, a technique which became popular in early radio broadcasting. He illuminated the microbe ... with two different wavelenghts of the same ultraviolet light frequency which resonated with the spectral signature of the microbe.

"These two wavelengths produced interference where they merged. The interference was, in effect, a third, longer wave which fell into the visible portion of the electromagnetic spectrum. This was how Rife made microbes visible without killing them, a feat which today's electron microscope cannot duplicate.

"By this time, Rife was so far ahead of his colleagues of the 1930's (!), that they could not comprehend what he was doing without actually traveling to San Diego to Rife's laboratory to look through his Virus Microscope for themselves. And many of them did exactly that."

"A Brief History of Dr. Royal Raymond Rife"
at website quantumbalancing.com
(This website has many good photos of
Rife, his microscopes, and news articles.)

"The microscope perfected by Dr. Rife after 18 years of experimentation accomplished what most physicists believed was impossible. It magnified to 20,000 or 30,000 times, still preserving the image in its true form and allowing it to be seen with the appearance of depth. It also revealed to the eye unstained cultures through the use of polarizing light and a monochromatic (one color) beam, thus making it possible to study living organisms." (Underlining added.)

"Microscope Magnifies to 31,000 Times"
Associated Press, September 22, 1933

"Rife began as a research pathologist. A medical crusader of the highest qualification, his was a heart filled with but one goal: the eradication of disease. Rife recognized first and foremost that successful medicine relies on vision, on light. What we cannot see, we cannot battle ... Therefore, his first quest was to secure a vastly improved system of microscopy. Once he could see, once all could see, then the pursuit of knowledge could move forward ... The creation of a supermicroscope would run counter to every physical law and restriction of the previous two centuries ... Rife succeeded in breaking the vision barrier." (Underlining added.)

Gerry Vassilatos
Lost Science

"So when you get light in the same range or a corresponding range, it will cause these microorganisms to fluoresce. This is something that people hadn't really done before, or since. Use monochromatic light to investigate micro-organisms and determine a species' specificity, you know, a specific species of micro-organism. One of the other working principles about it (Rife's microscope) was that the way that it channels the light never allows its beams of light to cross over themselves and create diffusion of light. So you continue to have your resolution. No matter how far you take the light path, you are not losing resolution. The Universal Microsocpe was a revolutionary breakthrough in optics altogether and it's a very simple principle that allows it to actually work. It's amazing that no one had discovered it before because it isn't really outside the technology that we've got at all. It's a fairly simple technology." (Underlining added.)

Michael Coyle, Ph.D., Microscopy
"The Rise and Fall of a Scientific Genius" (video) by Shawn Montgomery

"Can bacteria, viruses, and cancer cells be destroyed by resonance?" Question asked from biology.stackexchange.com. February 12, 2016.

Answered by Chris on August 19, 2017. Underlining added to Chris's answer.

"The answer is yes, of course you can kill microbes with resonant frequency(s) ... every form/organism in Creation and each sub-system of each form/organism has its own unique energy signature or resonant frequency.

"Nature has established all the parameters to this phenomenon. Each form emits its own energy frequency or 'energy signature.' When you feed a form its own energy signature, resonance occurs and energy is then absorbed rather than passing through or around -- a standing wave of energy is formed when resonance occurs. When you feed a form its matching energy at an amplitude that exceeds its natural emission level, the standing wave expands exponentially to a point where nature and Natural Law determines the energy must disperse lest it become disruptive to Nature itself. This dispersal of the energy is invariably disruptive to the form.

"We are talking about the natural electrostatic laws of resonant energy here. Very basic science. Very reliable. Very effective. If you want to know the full story and effectiveness of this technology, research Royal Rife."

"Using a simple electromagnetic wave is probably not sufficient. Dr. Rife found that using a wave that is emitted by a gas (within a glass tube) that has been excited by radio frequency energy – that particular wave that is emanated from that tube is a wave that is acceptable to the tissues of the body, for whatever reason, and it will penetrate deep within the body, and can be used to selectively oscillate those things that the (treating) *doctor ... chose to oscillate, and leave everything else alone in the body.*

"And that's the wonder of it all – that you have this selective scalpel-like effect using resonance. It's specific. It leaves everything else alone ... It's really quite an amazing, wondrous feat."

James Bare, D.C. interviewed in Shawn Montgomery's *The Rise and Fall of a Scientific Genius* (2004)

"Rife initially found that he could use specific electro-magnetic frequencies for killing bacteria and viruses without damaging the surrounding tissues. His machine used the law of sympathetic resonance. The law of sympathetic resonance says if there are two similar objects, and one of them begins to vibrate, the other will begin to vibrate too, even when they are not touching ... think of two identical tuning forks. If you tap either of them, the other will begin to vibrate in sympathy ... another example ... Ella Fitzgerald, the amazing singer who could strike a high note and shatter a crystal glass ... The glass shattered because of sympathetic resonance.

"This law was the basis of Rife's ability to destroy disease-producing organisms ... He built his Rife Machine to transmit the signal that would make microbes vibrate. By intensifying the signal for distance, he was able to shatter any microbe, just like Ella Fitzgerald's glass."

"Royal Raymond Rife" by Barbara Minton at tbyil.com

"Having invented the scope and come up with a new thing, he next reasoned that if he could illuminate a microorganism with a single frequency and cause it to resonate, then he should be able to turn that principle around and find some electromagnetic frequencies which could be redirected into living organisms to cause the disappearance of these organisms which are associated with diseases. And that is what he did!

Energetic Processes (2002, page 231) by Peter Moscow

Dr. Ronald R. Cowden was Emeritus Professor of Biophysics at the East Tennessee State University Medical School. He was also co-author of *Advances in Microscopy*, and an expert on 1930's optical materials! He examined the Rife Universal Microscope and planned to write an article for a science journal once it was again working. But a white collar crook interferred, using a $200,000 financing scam and fake restoration of the Universal as a prelude to STEALING it! The crook then swindled a patent on Rife's design principles. This con artist, aided by accomplices, caused a lasting setback for society. He prevented Dr. Cowden from demolishing the anti-Rife lies of corrupt interests and entry of bioelectric healing into medical school classrooms! Still, awareness of biophysics continues to grow – despite schemes by thieves.

"Rife machines work on the principle of RESONANCE which is very well known in physics. Everything in the universe has a natural resonant frequency which will cause it to vibrate. We've all seen videos where a singer can shatter a crystal glass if they produce just the right pitch, with a loud enough volume, for a long enough time ...

"Like wine glasses, microorganisms such as bacteria, viruses, etc. also have a natural resonance frequency that will cause them to vibrate. Rife machines use this principle of resonance to cause microorganisms to vibrate long enough and hard enough to self-destruct. Since the physical structure of each type of bacteria, virus, etc. is different, each type has its own unique resonant frequency. Thus, it is possible to kill one specific microorganism without damaging any other organisms or surrounding tissue. This approach to killing harmful microorganisms was pioneered by a man named Royal Raymond Rife." (Underlining added.)

"Rife Machine Primer --
How Do Rife Machines Work?"
December 14, 2018 at gurahq.com

"Dr. Rife's legacy exists in the estimated 400,000 frequency devices that are presently in use in the USA. The science foundation for the utilization, application, understanding and further development of electrical, magnetic, electromagnetic and acoustic-based frequency devices is very solid. Application of these principles to treatment has yielded empirical outcomes and results which are so common as to make the use of frequency devices a growing world wide phenomenon.

"Health care in the 21st century is going to be based upon the discoveries of the 20th century mixed with the knowledge learned in the new century. The old model of biochemical treatment will survive in very modified forms. New medications will be developed that interact specifically with pulsed electromagnetic fields." (Underlining added.)

"Royal Raymond Rife's Legacy" by James Bare
Conference on Future Energy, Washington, D.C.
October 9-10, 2009

"In the 1930s, a researcher by the name of Royal Raymond Rife made what should have become known as one of the most important discoveries of all time. Rife developed what was the most powerful and revolutionary medical microscope of all time ... using this microscope he saw things that no man had seen before ... he found that every organism responded to one frequency and that specific frequency would then cause the destruction of that organism. When he found the right frequency, it would just explode and die. Normal human cells were unaffected by these electromagnetic frequencies. The implications of this were profound. He had found a way to destroy bacteria and viruses and other disease-causing organisms without harming normal human cells. Even more important, Rife managed to find a way to selectively kill bacteria and viruses inside a human body." (Underlining added.)

Revolution of the Heart (2013) by Michel LeRoux

"With a live bacterial culture under the microscope, Rife would turn on a frequency device, known as Rife Beam Ray, that produced an electromagnetic field tuned to this (empirically derived) MOR frequency. Within moments of his turning on the field and hitting the correct frequency, all the bacteria would instantly stop moving and die. He found that he could utilize the Rife Beam Ray on people who were infected with a specific bacteria of vibratory resonance. Rife could destroy bacteria or viruses as easily as shattering a wine glass by producing its resonant note." (Underlining added.)

Vibrational Medicine (2001) by Richard Gerber, M.D.

"In October 1936, Dr. Ernest Walker of the Hooper Medical Foundation in San Francisco wrote a letter to Royal Rife after examining the results of one of Rife's experiments. Dr. Walker's words:

"The copy of the results of your test of the Rife ray on typhoid organisms would appear to estabish conclusively its efficiency to kill these organisms in the tissues. If the Ray should prove equally efficient in killing other micro-organisms, it would be the greatest discovery in the history of therapeutic medicine." (Underlining added.)

"Although frequency equipment has been substantially modified and redesigned since Rife's colleagues treated people in the 1930s, 40s, and 50s, the basic principles of how the devices work -- pathogenic destruction through resonance -- remains the same. There are now hundreds of companies, on every continent of the globe, selling frequency therapy units to address all types of disease ... widespread use of frequency therapy, including Rife's technology, promises to change the way medicine is practiced." (Underlining added.)

The Rife Handbook of Frequency Therapy by Nenah Sylver, Ph.D.

"In this fifteen year search, we found three original Rife machines and fully tested them. By doing this, we were able to find out how they really worked and the frequencies they used ... we found that almost all the so-called 'Rife Machines' sold on the market today do not use Dr. Rife's correct frequencies and cannot produce them with their low frequency equipment. Almost everyone is using the wrong frequencies.

"The most effective machine ever built was the Rife Ray #5 or Beam Ray Clinical instrument ... It was Dr. Rife's engineer Philip Hoyland who built this Beam Ray Clinical instrument ... It worked on harmonic sidebands and only worked on the two frequency method." (Underlining added.)

A History of Rife's instruments and Frequencies by Jeff Garff

"I regard energy medicine as profound. Energy medicine would be the talk of the day if Royal Rife's technology hadn't been shut down 80 years ago."

Steven A. Levine, Ph.D., molecular geneticist, *Townsend Letter* October 2016

"A noted cancer specialist in Boston said he believed that if some simple and inexpensive replacement for chemotherapy for the treatment of cancer were found tomorrow, all U.S. medical schools would teeter on the verge of bankruptcy, so integral a part of their hospital revenues is oncology, the medical specialty of cancer treatment." (Underlining added.)

Target Cancer by Edward J. Sylvester, professor at Cronkite School of Journalism, Arizona State University, and author of 5 books on medical research.

"The emergence of ... chemotherapy during the years following World War II was part of a new industrial medical complex that acted ruthlessly to eliminate competition in cancer treatment. Gradually, the public is waking up to the massive waste of taxpayer dollars on basic research and toxic cancer treatment that has led to few advances in survival rates ... millions of cancer patients have died because profits have been put before people." (Underlining added.)

"Suppression, Bias, and Selection in Science" by David J. Hess, Ph.D.
Accountability in Research, Vol. 6, website bmartin.cc/pub.

"In the United States, economic interests masquerade as therapeutic regimens and scientific concern. Their goal is to own and completely control a disease -- cancer ... and to quash competition (meaning alternative approaches), so as to maintain a marketplace monopoly.

"The financial interests of drug companies ... and others in what is known as the Cancer Establishment have eclipsed the integrity of the Hippocratic Oath; money and politics have proclaimed conventional approaches as scientifically validated and therefore mandated by law. The terrible flaw in this convenient financial setup is that the profits that flow to the cancer establishment are derived from human lives lost to cancer because successful alternative approaches are outlawed and unreported.

"To the cancer establishment, a cancer patient is a profit center. The actual clinical and scientific evidence does not support the claims of the cancer industry. Conventional cancer treatments are in place as the law of the land because they pay, not heal, the best." (Underlining Added.)

Alternative Medicine: The Definitive Guide to Cancer
by John Diamond, M.D. and Lee Cowden, M.D.
alternativemedicine.com

"Historically, all of the agencies involved in the war on cancer have lied about the nature of alternatives. Tests were performed only under duress (because the Congress insisted) and these tests were at best ill-conceived and at worst marked by outright fraud. The NCI, along with its police partner, the FDA, is the great roadblock to the examination of promising new ways of treating cancer."

Ralph Moss, Ph.D. testimony before Congress in 1998

"Eight years ago he began hunting the viruses with his microscope ... One of these previously undiscovered organisms, the scientist said, was that which is found in human carcinoma, or cancer.

"He saw on the slide a number of moving red-purple granules, the tiniest bits of microscopic life ever seen, only one-twentieth of a micron in length, so tiny that 500,000 of them placed end to end would span only the length of an inch on a ruler, he reported." (Underlining added.)

"Cancer Blow Seen After 18-year Toil by Rife"
by Newall Jones
San Diego Evening Tribune May 6, 1938

"Each kind of granule ... has ... under polarized light -- a distinctive color of its own, thereby enabling bacteriologists to diagnose germ-diseases by the color of the germs. Bacilli may thus be studied by their light, exactly as astronomers study moons, suns and other stars by the light which comes from them through telescopes. The bacilli studied are living ones, not corpses killed by stains.

"So extraordinary are these statements that scientists generally would regard them as visionary, or scientifically impossible, if they were not vouched for by such distinguished authorities ... The physicists and astronomers with whom I have discussed the matter are not yet convinced ... The absolute limit beyond which microscopes cannot go has been defined in these words, 'any object smaller than half of the wavelength of the light by which it is illuminated cannot be seen in its true form and size owing to diffraction.'

"On the other hand, this is a new kind of magnifier, and the laws governing microscopes may not apply to it ... 250 scientists present ... the impression prevailed that Dr. Rife, a 44-year (old) 'wizard' ... has developed an instrument that may revolutionize laboratory methods and enable bacteriologists like Dr. Kendall, to identify the germs that produce 50 diseases whose cause are unknown ... then to find ways and means to immunize mankind against them."

"The Wonderwork of 1931" by Ransom Sutton
Los Angeles Times Magazine December 27, 1931

"Despite widespread acceptance of Pasteur's germ theory, one germ for each disease, there were enough scientists who accepted pleomorphic theory of microbial organisms changing from helpful, benign, to pathogenic according to their immediate organic environments, or inner terrain.

"Later in the 20th century, circa 1930, a brilliant scientist named Royal Rife created what he called the Universal Microscope, a large complex instrument that was capable of magnifying even viruses. He was able to report microbial changes of form and size, often up to 16 phases of transition within the same microbe. Those of the pleomorphic persuasion were thrilled to witness proof of their beliefs with Rife's microscopic wizardry."

"Could There Be Something Wrong With The Germ Theory?
by Paul Fassa at vaccineimpact.com

"Dr. Rife developed equipment to apply frequencies. Since that time, various types of effective frequency devices have been produced. Hundreds of cancer patients have recovered without the benefits of surgery, chemotherapy or radiation ... many other conditions have yielded to frequency therapies. A woman had cancer in her right breast, right lung and in her right shoulder and ribs. Her right arm hung limp. She was heavily medicated for pain, and could not eat or keep supplements down due to nausea. Her husband decided to administer frequencies for six hours a day (not recommended). In a week she was able to stop her medications and she could take supplements and eat. After one month, cancer was no longer detectable, and she had use of her arm again."

Richard Lloyd, Ph.D., from *The Rife Handbook* by Nenah Sylver, Ph.D.

"... there is clinical evidence that ... radiotherapy EMF ... can cause therapeutic response in patients with cancerous states. The discovery is due to historical work ... in particular that of Rife ... In the first days of October 2013, the patient E.S. purchased the new apparatus. He began his treatment ... on October 04 ... the conclusion of this unique study is that a non-invasive bio-electromagnetic treatment ... for two months caused a disappearance of the patient's tumor ... constituting victory over the pancreatic cancer."

"Is Victory over Pancreatic Cancer Possible, with the Help of Tuned Non-Invasive Physiotherapy?" by Pierre Le Chapellier & Badri Matta, *Journal of Cancer Therapy*, Vol. 5, No. 5, 2014

"Under the universal microscope disease organisms such as those of tuberculosis, cancer, sarcoma, streptococcus, typhoid, staphylococcus ... and others may be observed to succumb when exposed to certain lethal frequencies peculiar to each individual organism, and directed upon them by rays covering a wide range of waves ... It should be emphasized that invariably the same organisms refract the same colors when stained by means of the monochromatic beam of illumination on the universal microscope.

"The virus of the *Bacillus typhosus* is always a turquoise blue, the *Bacillus coli* always mahogany colored, the *Mycobacterium leprae* always an emerald green, the virus of cancer always a purplish red, and so on." (Underlining added.)

"The New Microscopes" by R. E. Seidel and M. Elizabeth Winter
Annual Report of the Smithsonian Institute 1944

"We sincerely believe ... that BX in the primary cause of cancer ... We have used Koch's postulates in our methods of recovery ... this has been repeated hundreds of times proving to our own satisfaction that BX ... is the cause of malignancy." (Underlining added.)

History of the Development of a Successful Cure for Cancer
by Royal R. Rife (1953)

"Dr. Couche took Commander Benjamin Harrison's wife. She had a breast carcinoma. The lower half of the breast was ... eaten away and she suffered intense agaony all of the time. But she didn't want to have it operated on because her husband had told her that if she was ever operated on, she would die ... because of the metastasizing of the operation and spreading it out in the blood stream. Well, he (Dr. Couche using his own Rife instrument) healed her up perfectly and her breasts took on the normal shape ... When she realized that she had two normal breasts again, it was to her a most marvelous thing." (Underlining added.)

"John Crane Interviews Ben Cullen:
October 15, 1950, Answers 14 & 15"
website Rifevideos.com

Why Rife's Therapy Won't Be Allowed

Ralph Moss, Ph.D. has written 13 books and made three film documentaries on cancer. He was a founding advisor to the NIH Office of Alternative Medicine, a board member of the Cancer Prevention Coalition, and active in evaluating alternative cancer therapies. He is the author of *The Cancer Industry* and also *Questioning Chemotherapy.* Here he describes his experience at the edges of the "establishment" cancer world. (Underlining Added.)

"I was on the alternative medicine program advisory council ... And the split was ... whether to take the most controversial things that the public was most interested in and evaluate those things fairly honestly and without prejudice ... the other people .. believed what should happen is the money .. should go to the most prestigious university ... studies that were periperal to the controversial treatments ... the controversial treatments never happened.

"... all these things that were enormously interesting to the public were completely off limits in terms of the academic medical establishment ... one hundred and two different treatments ... in cancer therapy shrunk down ... until it became acupuncture and massage ... couldn't touch anything that anybody in the establishnent of any importance had ever said anything negative about."

"... the kiss of death. And they can do that .. but you'll never get to be a player in terms of setting the policy or being able to move the direction. The only way you can influence this behemoth is to mobilize public opinion. That's the only power that you have, this is my experience. And that's unfair .. unfair to the patients ... asking cancer patients to fight for freedom of choice.

"So it's a very difficult situation because this juggernaut rolls on ... And there's an abundance of evidence that there's a better outcome ... and you're ignored. I hear horror story after horror story about how people are treated by the oncologist. The oncologists don't want others to poach on what they consider their field. They want to have the monopoly as a group.

"... there's a whole elaborate structure that's been created that involves hundreds of thousands of people. This is not a little cabal. This is a huge profession, gigantic profession. Their meetings have twenty-five thousand people for the ASCO meeting ... American Society for Clinical Oncology."

"It reminds me a little bit of the church in the late Middle Ages."

Moss Reports #22 **at website Connorsclinic.com**

Rife's Frequencies

These are the most accurate M.O.R.s known. They were presented in Chapter 13 of Jeff Garff's "A History of Rife's instruments and Frequencies" which can be read at rifevideos.com. If your "Rife" Machine cannot deliver these radio frequencies, you don't have a true Rife Machine.

Actinomycosis (Streptothrix)	191,803 Hz
Anthrax	139,200 Hz
B. Coli (Rod Form)	416,510 Hz
B. Coli (Filterable Virus)	769,035 Hz
BX (Cancer Carcinoma)	1,607,450 Hz
BY (Cancer Sarcoma)	1,529,520 Hz
Gonorrhea	233,000 Hz
Spinal Meningitis	426,862 Hz
Staphylococcus Pyogenes Aureaus	477,660 Hz
Staphylococcus Pyogenes Albus	549,070 Hz
Streptococcus Pyogenes	719,150 Hz
Syphilis	788,700 Hz
Tetanus	234,000 Hz
Tuberculosis (Rod)	369,433 Hz
Tuberculosis (Virus)	769,000 Hz
Typhoid Fever (Rod)	759,450 Hz
Typhoid Fever (Virus)	1,445,180 Hz

These are Royal Rife's reliable, scientifically proved frequencies for the microbial causes of many diseases. A person with a quality Rife frequency instrument may be cured by using the appropriate frequency for a specific disease. Allow a few days intervals between treatments. "This gives the lymphatic system an opportunity to absorb and cast off the toxic condition which is produced by the devitalized dead particles" (Royal Rife).

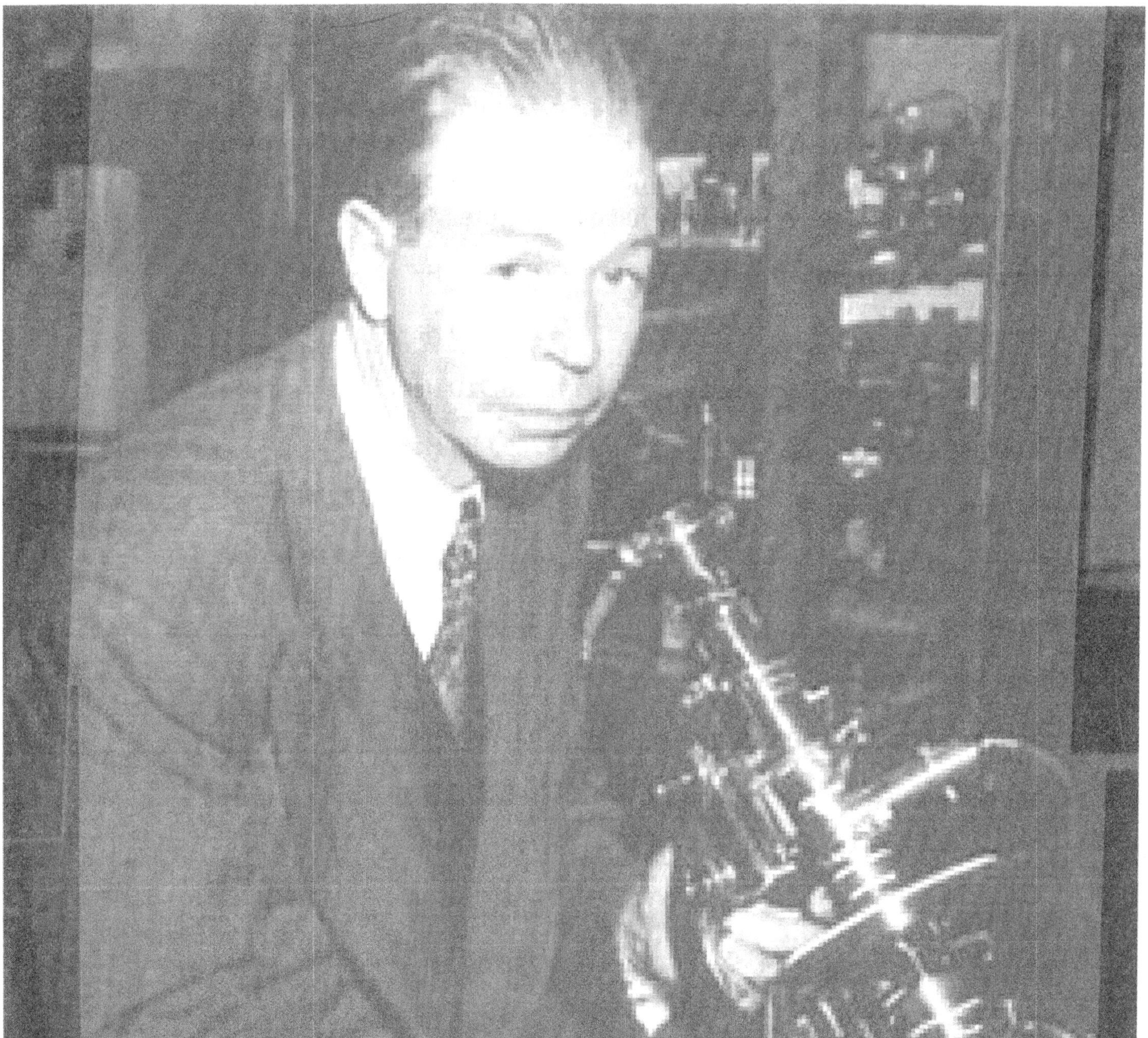

Royal Rife left us these words, spoken at his funeral for him:

"I hope I have helped humanity some. I am just an ordinary man, doing the best he can. We are all here to do our part. Each has a purpose as he lives it and thinks it. The most important thing I ever did was build a microscope."

The Rife Universal Microscope

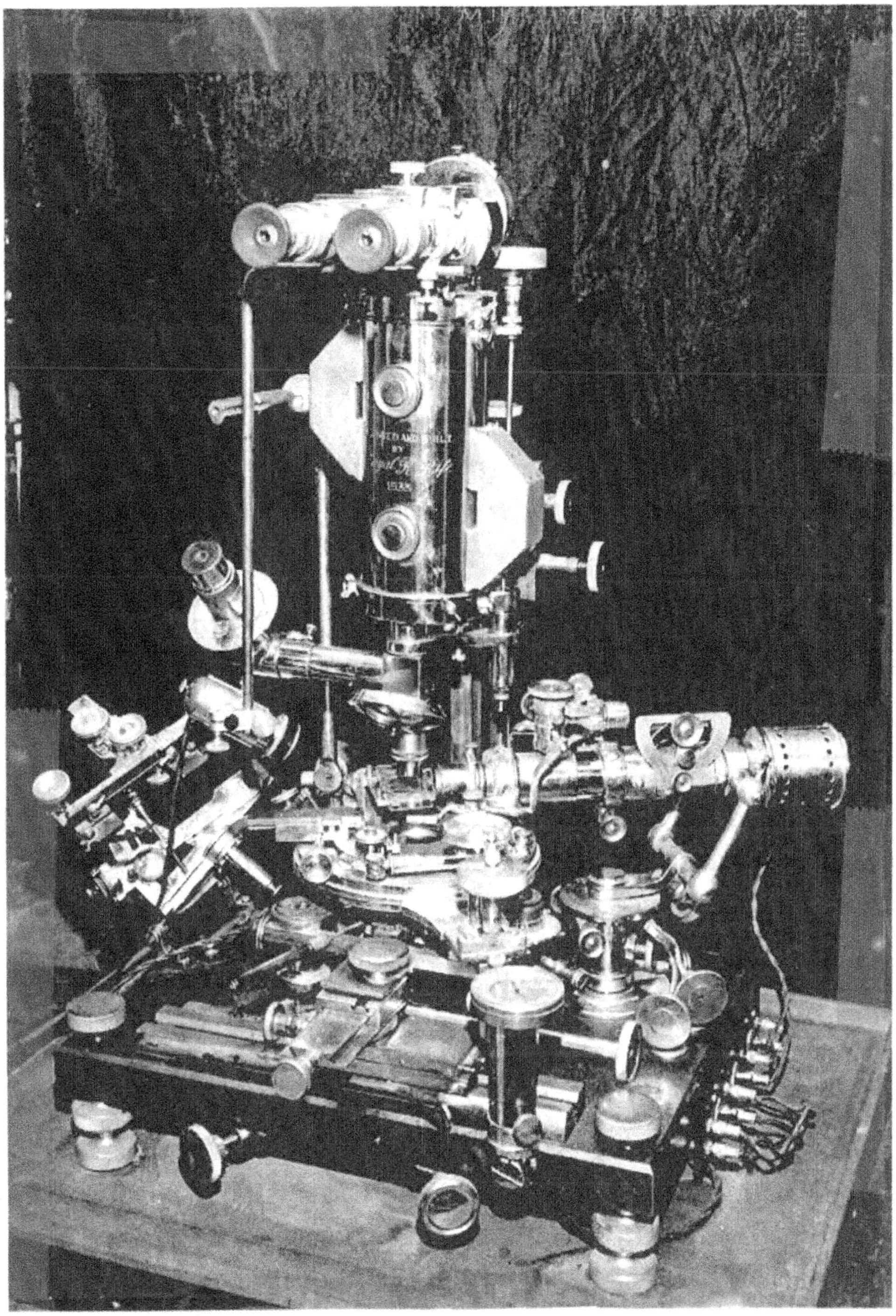

This is the most valuable microscope in the world. Most valuable in the sense of its benefit to society -- because this microscope enabled the oscillatory rates of the microbe causes of humanity's most deadly diseases to be determined. Which will lead to these pathogens being painlessly, noninvasively destroyed through "resonance." Its optical principles and design will change the world. It deserves to be displayed in a museum -- or many museums -- so the public can view this science "masterpiece" which, in time, will elevate the health of people across the globe.

Dr. James B. Couche, M.D. Describes A Fantastic Case

"Now the Rife machine had covered a band of frequencies, each frequency having a specific germ attached to it. And I had a list of the frequencies that had been demonstrated by Dr. Rife and others in their experimental work of what frequency would kill turberculosis, the virus, and what frequency the rod (bacteria) for another.

"Each one of the different germs had its frequency worked out ... Knowing the frequency for tuberculosis, I turned on the machine ... knowing it couldn't hurt her ... So I gave her what the machine had at that distance, not touching her.

"So she came back the next morning ... All the soreness gone. 'Oh nonsense,' I said. 'Get on the table.' Sure enough, on the table, there wasn't a sign of the lump swelling. And I began punching it. 'I don't mind,' she said. 'It's all right. It's all gone. No soreness there at all.'

"And I might say at this time I've seen her for many years since. *Well, that is a startling case because I practically instantly cured her of tuberculosis. And it was a most outstanding condition.*

"I went to England and over there I introduced the machine to those people over there. Or told them about the machine." (Underlining added for emphasis.)

****

In 1938-1939, when Henry Siner (Rife's Lab Assistant) brought Rife's smaller #4 microscope to London, he gave a demonstration to the President of the Royal Microscopical Society, In the CD #14 of taped interviews ("The Rife Tapes), Siner describes the moment when the prominent British microscopist saw a new world. Siner recalled:

"I met some of the most outstanding people in Europe. President of the Microscopical Society ... showed him hanging drops and culture (under the microscope). He focused it himself. Objective lens and optic lens. He was very competent. Remember, this man was one of the great men in microscopes in Europe. 'I don't believe it,' he said. 'I've done it myself, but I don't believe it.' " World War II prevented a global sales effort from London of Rife machines through a Rife-British partnership. Today's medicine would have been forever advanced to an exalted level.

3 Quality DVDs Will Enable People To See And Hear Royal Rife In An Informative And Beautiful Manner

These 3 videos are available from various sources. By purchasing one or more of them, you will own a look at a lost history which you can share with family, friends, and other associates -- enabling them to quickly learn of Royal Rife's discoveries and inventions.

The beauty of seeing the man alongside visuals which explain the critical elements of his science and vibrational healing means people do not have to read long books. In an hour or two, they can leap into a "place" where they understand the essential genius who brought the world astounding knowledge about (1) the micro world and (2) disease processes. This will also prepare them for the kind of "new" medicine that will become available as Americans make a transition to electro-medicine from chemo medicine! These 3 videos provide wonderful starting places for anyone who knows nothing about Royal Rife to grasp the full heroic impact of what Royal Rife accomplished.

So, having one or more of these three videos in your residence can enable you to introduce others to a new way to gain optimum health for an entire lifetime. Royal Rife's discoveries will be with us for a long time. Here are the 3 very fine videos about RRR. All are highly recommended.

The Royal Rife Story

Royal Rife In His Own Words

The Rise and Fall of A Scientific Genius:
The Forgotten Story of Royal Raymond Rife

"In every culture and in every medical tradition before ours, healing was accomplished by moving energy."

Albert Szent-Gyorgyi, Nobel Prize Winner for Medicine, 1937

"In Rife's era, it was proven that his frequency devices disable microbes that made humans and animals sick. But we now know that selected frequencies can regenerate tissue ... The body is composed of EM radiations. It emits EM waves and responds to EM waves. All biological functions correspond to electromagnetic phenomena. The electromagnetic energies that exist in living tissue are extremely potent. When you target a living cell with the precise frequency that it needs, it will respond favorably, and health can be restored in an amazingly short period of time.

"The health restoration effects of correctly applied energetics cannot be underestimated. As with any modality, one must be careful when using frequencies ... However, as those who have benefited from electromagnetic therapies can attest, the correct energies, properly used, can be an integral part of one's wellness protocol. Electromedicine and sound are the healing of the future." (Underlining Added.)

"Healing With Electromedicine and Sound Therapies"
by Nenah Sylver, Ph.D. at website nenahsylver.com

"Royal Rife was an American inventor who created the Universal Microscope. His contributions along with that of others offer alternatives and directions for study that might not have ever been considered were it not for his work. Rife's microscope allowed the real time viewing of live specimens at resolutions never before allowed.

"Society is continuously evolving and gaining new knowledge and power. The next step in the future of medicine is vitalizing energy and recharging our bodies. With this insight of the body, society can only grow further and advance in higher levels of understanding. The works of Rife, Galvani, Maxwell, Faraday and Tesla have built the foundations to a whole new world that we are barely entering ... We need to dwell on what our bodies were created around and revitalize our bio-energy fields." (Underlining Added.)

Physicist Auguste Meessen's Closing Judgment

"Rife discovered already about 100 years ago that bacteria and nanobacteria can be destroyed by resonance ... He did then prove that some of them are present in cancer tissue and that after being cultured, they do cause cancer. He determined the resonant frequency for targeted destruction of microbes. Those values were confirmed by two collaborators, using different equipment.

"The efficiency of his method for healing cancer was clinically tested, but even these results were declared to be bogus since they required modifying cherished postulates. For those who had the power to crush Rife, it did not matter that the reported results might be true ... all traces of his achievements were eradicated from official medical record. That was *profoundly unjust, truly antiscientific and detrimental* for the worldwide health system.

"We solved the basic scientific puzzle with mathematical rigor by considering the spikes of viruses, as well as pili of bacteria and nanobacteria ...The theory is experimentally confirmed and leaves no rational reason to negate the possibility of targeted destruction of microbes.

"The Coronavirus pandemic and its social implications should make everyone attentive to existence of a biophysical method that differs from the usual biochemical one, but is *effective, secure and rapidly adoptable*.

"There is also rising evidence that our precious arsenal of antibiotics is endangered. Multiple antibacterial resistances are increasing. The U.S. Centers for Disease Control concluded ... that 'coordinated effort to implement new politics, renew research efforts, and pursue steps to manage the crisis are greatly needed.' This was thought to 'require considerable investment,' but that is not true for Rife's method. it only required to change habits of thought.

"... dogmatism and concentration of power endanger scientific progress by blocking freedom of thought. Rife made a great discovery. We did only explain why apparently unbelievable, but observed facts are true."

Rife's Method of Healing Disease Deserves Support

A great crime was committed when Rife's clinically-proven therapy of curing cancer and other diseases through resonance destruction of a disease's microbial cause was suppressed by "official medicine" protecting their own financial interests. At the expense of the public's health! People who worked for U.S. government agencies, AMA officials, private cancer charities, and especially pharma formed a powerful combination to prevent this biophysics technology from being honestly investigated and widely developed. The historical evidence of this organized prohibition against a momentous scientific discovery is sufficiently strong to conclude that it is part of a larger pattern and corrupt enterprise imposed by the medical monopoly on the American people.

"... cancer research and its treatment using chemo, radiation and surgery has become a very lucrative business despite the dismal success record.

"... Numerous promising cures continue to be actively suppressed to protect the vested interests of various branches of the medical monopoly, including its regulators which all appear to be in bed together in this conspiracy of suppression and silence.

"The existing approach of continuing with long term dependence on costly artificial drugs with all their indeterminate and frequently fatal side effects must be stopped if our health care system is to return to some measure of sanity.

"... the real blame for this horrendous miscarriage of professional ethics rests entirely with the upper level power brokers who perpetuate the symptomatic focus of modern medicine for entirely selfish reasons, using corrupt regulatory practices to advance their monopolistic purposes, fleecing the public with exhorbitant healthcare costs and providing woefully inadequate services, all the while padding their bank vaults with obscene levels of 'ill-gotten gain'.

"... It is an absolute travesty that in so called democratic nations priding themselves on freedom, that totalitarian agencies such as these can prevent terminally ill cancer patients from even accessing information, let alone electing for treatments of their own choice." (Underlining added.)

Excerpts from the Introduction to *Cancer Cures and Cover-Ups: Political and Economic Corruption of Healthcare* (2006) by Mark Porringa. Entire Introduction available at website holimedex.com.

How NIH Elite Sabotage Alternative Therapies

From 1991 onward, there was an effort to finance research of alternative medicine through first the Office of Alternative Medicine (OAM) which became the National Center for Complementary and Alternative Medicine (NCCAM). Then National Center for Complementary and Integrative Health (NCCIH). For thirty-one years (1991-2022), they AVOIDED Royal Rife's incredible inventions and discoveries. The science bureaucrats shared anti-Rife groupthink within a dishonest system, so the public went out and got modern Rife devices and some obtained fanatastic cures! Did NCCIH get excited over professor Meessen's 2020 Biophysics confirmation of Rife's therapy? Nope. Silence tells so much.

Former Iowa Congressman Berkley Bedell served on an advisory committee of OAM for 8 years. He later recalled how the committee was unanimous in wanting to do field trials. "Send people out to check what was happening with alternative doctors around the world. And where those treatments appeared to be effective, to run trials to confirm or refute their effectiveness. But the NIH absolutely refused to do any checking of any of the alternative treatments." Congress's intent to honestly test alternative therapies was sabotaged by the science elite at NIH who serve Pharma profits and thus shield chemotherapy from being ended! The cost of patient deaths is a business expense.

In dealing with the institutional corruption of the National Cancer Institute (NCI), Dr. Robert Atkins wrote so clearly of the monumental betrayal of the public trust by government cancer officials that after 1988 -- when Dr. Atkins's book was a best seller -- there was no excuse for the press to avoid doing an investigation of the cancer holocaust's corrupt cause. Chemo killed, but its huge profits kept it from being replaced by safer therapies that worked!

"I find it hard to believe that officials of the National Cancer Institute, whose careers are devoted to knowing about cancer research, would be unaware. It is much more plausible that they are aware of what is going on and choose to pretend that it is not ... The entire concept of a biologic, nontoxic cancer therapy would signal the beginning of the end of the highly profitable chemotherapy industry ... there have already been many cancer cures, and all have been ruthlessly and systematically suppressed ... by the cancer establishment ... which profits so much from our profession-wide obsession with chemotherapy ... the damage done to the body by an unsuccessful course of chemotherapy is often so great that the patient's immune system never recovers significantly."

Dr. Atkins Health Revolution by Robert C. Atkins (1988)

A Word About Wikipedia's Distortions

Anyone who seeks information about Royal Rife by visiting Wikipedia's website will receive a deliberate distortion of Rife's inventions and important discoveries. Fortunately, Auguste Meessen's December 2020 article, "Virus Destruction by Resonance" that appeared in the *Journal of Modern Physics* means that serious scientists can now learn some of the physics laws and equations that confirm Rife's claims.

Throughout Wikipedia's hit job on Royal Rife's legacy, the reader will find clever ways of disparaging Rife's achievement. For instance, they start by using the American Medical Association (AMA) and the American Cancer Society (ACS) as credible authorities for dismissing Rife's real scientific discoveries! When it was the AMA boss Morris Fishbein who sought to steal ownership and control of Rife's resonance therapy in 1939, but who was rebuffed by the judge in the AMA's phony legal action! Why would any honest information source use a discredited institution with a glaring conflict-of-interest about science facts? It wouldn't. But a dishonest source like Wikipedia doing a hatchet job would!

James De Meo, Ph.D., offered this warning about "the suppression of new ideas and discoveries by unethical and repressive methods ... the authoritarian medical-academic power structure ... is similar to any other authoritarian hierarchical political or even military structure ... well-documented evidence of the conspiratorial collusion between pharmacy companies, medical organizations and government agencies ... is generally directed at the suppression of non-allopathic MD health practitioners who tend to use more natural and inexpensive methods ... war against natural healing methods began in the 1930s and 1940s, and has continued since, carried forward by power and money motivations, to establish a medical monopoly on health care."

Linus Pauling (1901-1994) won the Nobel Prize for chemistry in 1954. Then Linus Pauling won the Nobel Peace Prize in 1962. Linus Pauling wrote the following in a letter to Ralph Moss, Ph.D. on October 24, 1979: *"I have read with great interest your book The Cancer Rebellion: Hope and Betrayal ... The revelations in this book about the ways in which the American people have been betrayed by the cancer establishment, the medical profession, and the government are shocking. Everyone should know that the 'War on cancer' is largely a fraud and that the National Cancer Institute and American Cancer Society are derelict in their duties to the people who support them."*

Notice how Wikipedia's language describes Rife's great discovery in a way that seems to imply it's a ridiculous science claim: "Rife reported that a 'beam ray' device of his invention could destroy microbial pathogens. Rife claimed to have documented a 'Mortal Oscillatory Rate" for various pathogenic organisms, and to be able to destroy the organism by vibrating them using radio waves of this particular frequency."

Wow. That really sounds silly, doesn't it? Until you allow a real physicist like Auguste Meessen to explain Rife's discovery. Meessen tells the truth:

"For those who had the power to crush Rife, it did not matter that the reported results might be true ... all traces of his achievements were eradicated from official medical records. That was *profoundly unjust, truly antiscientific and detrimental* for the worldwide health system."

"The theory is experimentally confirmed and leaves no rational reason to negate the possibility of targeted destruction of microbes ... Rife made a great discovery."

Wikipedia -- in its ignorance – tried to make a great science discovery seem absurd. But Rife's discovery will gain recognition and bring cures of deadly diseases to countless millions. If only Wikipedia had encouraged honest investigation instead of a stupid lie. Here's more Meessen truth:

"... the now available explanation should make it obvious that biophysical methods cannot be rejected anymore."

"It was a huge error to claim that the observed facts had to be bogus, without verifying, since it deprived humanity from use of a simple and secure method to fight sicknesses, plaques and even cancer."

"Rife discovered ... that bacteria and nanobacteria can be destroyed by resonance. Instead of emitting EM waves in all directions by means of an antenna like Hertz did and is usual for broadcasting, his system generated a local beam of EM waves."

"We solved the basic scientific puzzle with mathematical rigor by considering the spikes of viruses as well as pili of bacteria and nanobacteria can be set in forced oscillation. Nonlinear effects make the resonance stronger and sharper than the usual ones. This theory is experimentally confirmed ..."

The Rockefeller Medical Trust

"It all starts with John D. Rockefeller (1839-1937) who was an oil magnate, a robber baron, America's first billionaire, and a natural-born monopolist ... By the turn of the 20th century he controlled 90% of all oil refineries in the U.S. through his oil company, Standard Oil.

"At the same time ... scientists discovered 'petrochemicals' and the ability to create all kinds of chemicals from oils ... pharmaceutical drugs could be made from oil. This was a wonderful opportunity for Rockefeller who saw the ability to monopolize the oil, chemical and medical industries at the same time.

"Rockefeller ... went to his buddy Andrew Carnegie -- another plutocrat who made his money from monopolizing the steel industry -- who devised a scheme. They sent a man named Abraham Flexner to travel around the country and report on the state of medical colleges and hospitals ... This led to the Flexner Report which gave birth to modern medicine ... Based on this report, more than half of all medical colleges were soon closed. Homeopathy and natural medicines were mocked and demonized and doctors were even jailed.

"In a very short time, medical colleges were all streamlined and homogenized. All the students were learning the same thing, and medicine was all about patented drugs.

"So, now we are, 100 years later, churning out doctors who know nothing about the benefits of nutrition or herbs or any holistic practice. We have an entire system that is enslaved to corporations ... Why would there be real cures? This is a system founded by oligarths and plutocrats, not by doctors."

"How Rockefeller Founded Modern Medicine And Killed Natural Cures"
An Excerpt from Worldaffairs.blog on October 20, 2015

"The medical-drug cartel was summed up by J.W. Hodge, M.D. of Niagra Falls, N.Y. in these words: 'The medical monopoly or medical trust, euphemistically called the American Medical Association, is not merely the meanest monopoly ever organized, but the most arrogant, dangerous organization which ever managed a free people in this or any other age."

"The Truth About The Rockefeller Drug Empire" by Hans Ruesch, whale.to

"The Rockefeller-initiated medical cartel which revamped US medicine in the early 1900s has grown into an enormous bureaucracy comprising doctors, hospitals, support services and government regulators like the FDA, NIH and CDC, all working closely with Big Pharma to ensure their steadily increasing profits at the expense of Americans.

"Despite the efforts of the cartel to suppress cancer therapies, many have succeeded in actually curing thousands of terminal patients so that they can return to normal life.

"The Food and Drug Administration ... works hand in hand with the AMA using federal courts to prosecute natural therapies for the benefit of Big Pharma ... The revolving door between the Drug monoliths and the FDA is well known.

"With hundreds of billions of funds allocated, vast corruption abounds in scientific studies, peer reviews, fake test results and incentives for physicians to over-prescribe, all sanctioned by the Medical Cartel while ensuring Big Pharma receives the lion's share of the money.

"Those subjected to orthodox therapy without being given a choice are trapped in the Cancer Vortex with little chance of being cured."

Cancer Vortex (2014) by Kenneth V. Anton

Kenneth Anton's book (above) reveals the end product of National Cancer Institute "experts," aided by the corrupt programs of the "alternative medicine agency" (OAM, NCCAM, NCCIH). Along with the prosecution of physicians who dare offer natural, "unapproved" therapies that in some cases cure cancer. The evidence clearly shows institutional sabotage of therapies that were threats to the Drug Trust's profits and criminal malpractice. The antidote to this evil was offered on page 38 of this book – copying Germany's successful cancer program where physicians can legally offer something better! Be it Rife's "resonance" therapy or a dozen different therapies that have delivered real healing.

The evidence that a vast conspiracy exists to prevent the use of new discoveries and known alternative therapies in the treatment of cancer is overwhelming. It's time for a democracy to create a true healing system.

Cancer Quagmire: Profiteering, Deceit, Suppression

"... the NCI (National Cancer Institute), with enthusiastic support from the ACS (American Cancer Society) ... has effectively blocked funding for research and clinical trials on promising, non-toxic alternative cancer drugs for decades in favor of highly toxic and largely ineffective patented drugs developed by the multibillion dollar global cancer drug industry. Additionally, the cancer establishment has systematically harassed the proponents of non-toxic alternative cancer drugs."

The Politics of Cancer by Dr. Samuel Epstein

"The cancer industry tells us some of the most magnificent lies about the safety of toxic chemotherapy treatments and long-term survival rates related to this poisonous practice. Few doctors and scientists will put their reputations on the line to expose this fraudulent source of disease called a treatment.

"We will one day look back on the practice of 'cut, burn or poisoning' cancer as perhaps the most barbaric and one of the largest failures of mainstream medicine." (Underlining added.)

website dailyhealthpost.com

"Success of most chemotherapy is appalling ... There is no scientific evidence for its ability to extend in any appreciable way the lives of patients suffering from the most common organic cancer ... chemotherapy for malignancies too advanced for surgery, which accounts for 80% of all cancers, is a scientific wasteland." (Underlining added.)

Dr. Ulrich Abel, author of the classic global chemo study

"If cancer specialists were to admit publicly that chemotherapy is of limited usefulness and is often dangerous, the public might demand a radical change in direction toward unorthodox and nontoxic methods, and toward cancer prevention ... The use of chemotherapy is even advocated by those members of the estabishment who realize how ineffective and dangerous it can be."

Ralph Moss, Ph.D., noted cancer scholar

"A full-fledged crusade to suppress all real cures for disease would have to be launched to protect the pharmaceutical-centric system from any real competition. Recognizing that nobody would agree to take chemical drugs if cheaper, safer, and much more effective natural remedies were available, the medical oligarchy had to get busy knocking them out, one by one.

"One of the most tragic examples of post-Flexner Report medical cronyism is the persecution of Royal Raymond Rife. This distinguished scientist and inventor is credited ... with discovering that every disease microbe has its own electronic signature, and that the electronic signature can be neutralized or 'devitalized' in order to cure the disease the microbe causes.

"Rife's brilliant mind led him to embark on a much different scientific journey that would lead to some truly groundbreaking discoveries in the field of bioelectric medicine -- Rife's universal microscope allowed scientists to see ... live viruses and bacteria in true animated color profiles, and at magnification levels needed for advanced study.

"... electronic signatures ... got him thinking. What if customized frequencies could be developed for each known pathogen in order to destroy that pathogen, and possibly cure the particular disease associated with it? ... Rife learned that by identifying, isolating, and matching an ... organism's signature with electro-frequency energy, it was fully possible to cure diseases.

"This discovery was especially relevant with regard to cancer ... This newly found virus ... became the means through which he would identify a viable cure." (Underlining added.)

The Truth About Cancer: What You Need To Know
About Cancer's History by Ty M. Bolingen

"The Beam Ray ... became an unthinkable threat to established medicine. Objects began disappearing from Rife's lab on Alcott Street; photos and films of dwarf bacteria, notes, and records. A fire destroyed the Burnett lab in New Jersey, where researchers were about to announce success with the Beam Ray. In 1944, all the records at USC disappeared." (Underlining added.)

"Royal Raymond Rife: Into The Micro Beyond"
by Jeff Smith at *San Diego Reader* February 15, 2012

Summation

Here's the essence of this important change in direction for medicine. For 80+ years official medicine suppressed and censored a great science discovery -- the healing of any microbe-based disease by destroying the cause (virus, bacteria, nanobacteria, etc.) through resonance! (Without harming any other cells or organs in the patient's body!) Physics doing with certainty what chemistry medicine does so inconsistently. But Pharma and doctor interests were determined to keep such a therapy from disrupting "their empires." The so profitable medical drug practices. The AMA thus quashed the most unique, low-cost, efficient, and socially valuable therapy ever discovered.

It was a thorough interdiction of an alternative therapy validated by a successful clinical trial. Until 2020 when someone with impeccable physics credentials blew the whistle -- exposing medical authorities for suppressing and censoring an enormously important biophysics discovery that could bring the world momentous benefits in healing microbe-based diseases. In December 2020, this top physicist explained in the *Journal of Modern Physics* why the condemned biophysics method was actually a superior medical technique to cure ALL deadly diseases caused by microbes.

This physicist dared to write a 41-page *tour de force* article for the science community! It revealed the decades-long AMA-led endeavor to hide the power of resonance healing. The physicist provided lots of proof to silence the medical gatekeepers from continuing the suppression of Royal Rife's microscope and Royal Rife's discovery of how to reverse and cure microbe-caused diseases!

The physicist stated it was time to honor Royal Rife because "his scientific creativity and accomplished craftsmanship deserve recognition and respect. Rife discovered ... that bacteria and nanobacteria can be destroyed by resonance. Rife made a great discovery. This theory is experimentally confirmed and leaves no rational reason to negate the possibility of targeted destruction of microbes."

A great leap in healing is imminent – based on a switch from the biochemical monopoly to a dual system which include's Rife's biophysics therapy. As Gerry Vassilatos exclaimed in *Lost Science,* "The world potential of this (Rife's) system was staggering."

Dangerous Genius

Rife was "undeniably awe-inspiring." He came to show us something special. He deserved more help. Imagine what health tools we'd have today if the science community had encouraged him <u>from 1940 to 1970</u>! When "special interests" put the order out to suppress Rife's findings. And scientists were bribed and told to stop helping Dr. Rife. And when established institutions and health agencies ignored Dr. Rife and harassed his associates!

Our modern "experts" and research leaders should take note. Fresh ideas and approaches need to be honestly tested. What usually is being "officially" funded is often stupid, outdated, or meritless and based purely on a political payback. And still our government science potentates avoid and deny what Dr. Rife discovered and invented. History will be scornful.

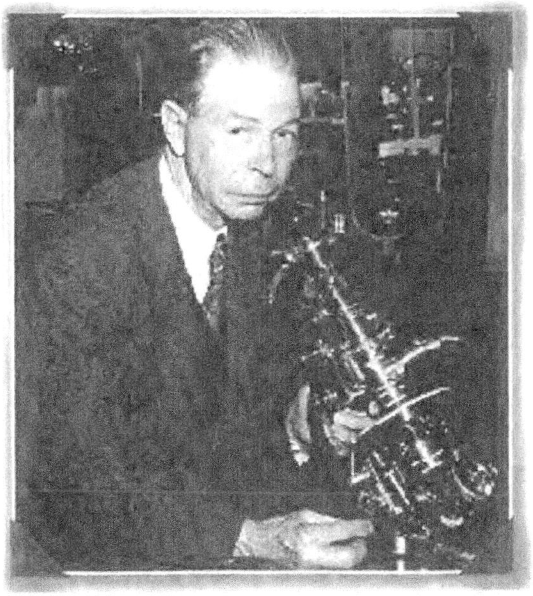

Royal Rife

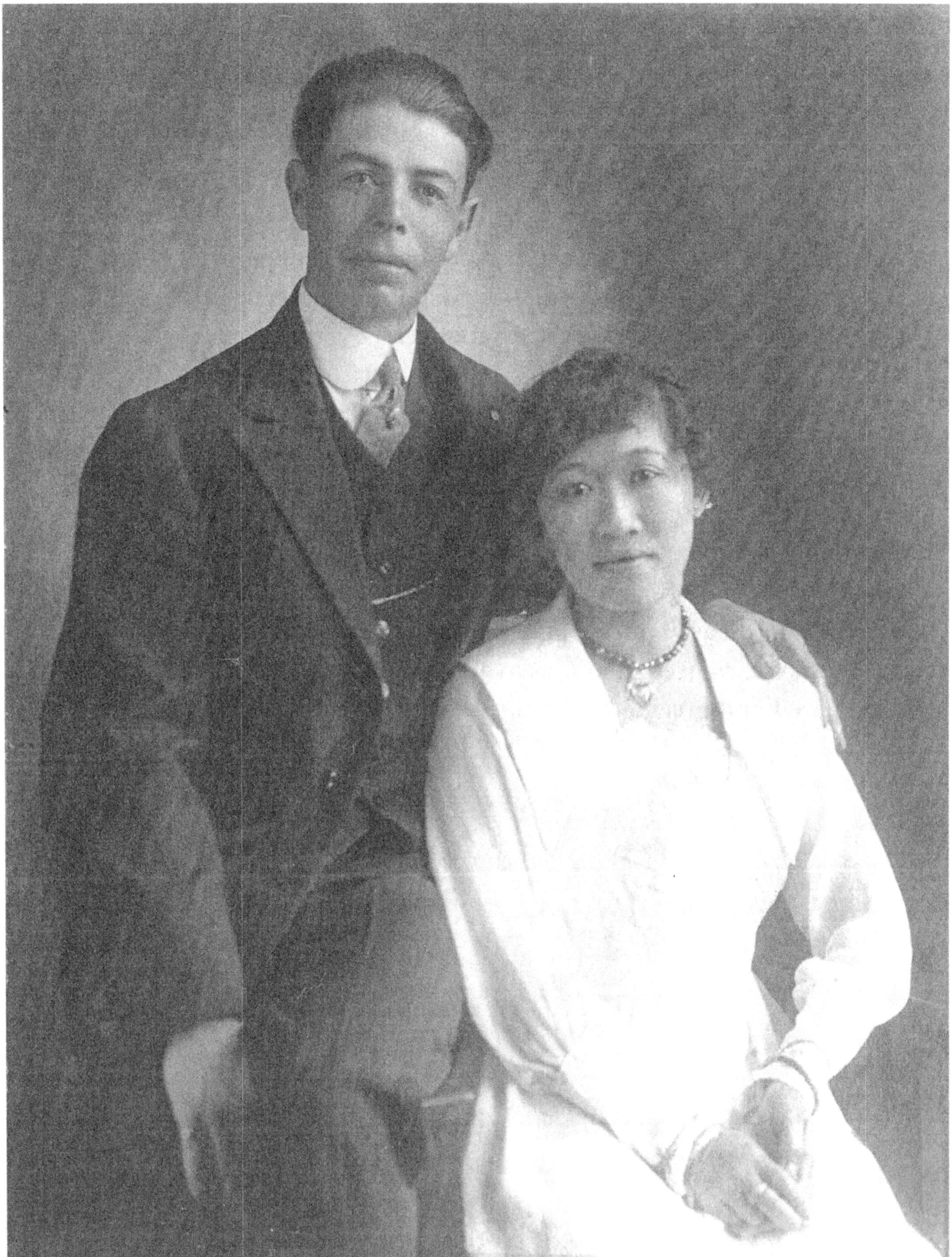

Royal and Mamie Rife

About The Author

Barry Lynes joined the U.S. army the week the Cuban Missile Crisis began. He later served at U.S. Army Europe Headquarters in Heidelberg, Germany and then Supreme Headquarters Allied Powers Europe (SHAPE) outside Paris, France. Following military service, he received a B.A. degree in English Literature from Boston University. A few years later, Lynes became an adviser to Italian film director Federico Fellini for the movie *Casanova*, a typical phantasmagoria Fellini magical cinema experience.

Several years afterwards while living in Washington, D.C., Lynes met and shared climate research with Christopher Bird, New York Times bestselling co-author of *The Secret Life of Plants.* Bird also wrote the article, "What Has Become Of The Rife Microscope?" which was published in *New Age* magazine in March 1976. This was the first article published after 30 years of organized medicine's suppression and censorship of <u>Royal Rife's amazing inventions and scientific discoveries</u>. Lynes's meeting with Christopher Bird led to John Crane – Rife's living partner – contacting Lynes about a book concerning Royal Rife, who had died in 1971.

Lynes subsequently authored the April 1987 book *The Cancer Cure That Worked – The Rife Report*, which initiated the "Rife Revival" of modern times. Florence Seibert, the Women's Hall of Fame scientist who discovered the TB skin test, endorsed *The Rife Report* by writing that it was "far superior to anything we scientists could write." Now, 36 years later, Lynes offers with the 2023 publication of *The New Royal Rife Book* what 3 1/2 decades of dedicated work by modern "Rifers" have produced -- a sophisticated knowledge about the future healing technology that Royal Rife's genius gave to humans everywhere.

Made in the USA
Monee, IL
19 September 2026

63557821R00050